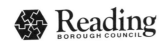

THE MEAT FIX

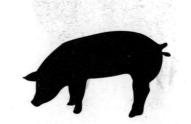

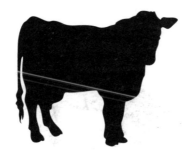

JOHN NICHOLSON

THE MEAT FIX

HOW A LIFETIME OF HEALTHY EATING NEARLY KILLED ME!

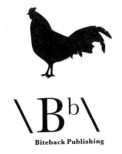

\B^b\
Biteback Publishing

First published in Great Britain in 2012 by
Biteback Publishing Ltd
Westminster Tower
3 Albert Embankment
London
SE1 7SP

ISBN 978-1-84954-139-8

10 9 8 7 6 5 4 3 2 1

A CIP catalogue record for this book is available from the British Library.

Set in Dolly and Naked
Cover design by Namkwan Cho

Printed and bound in Great Britain by
CPI Group (UK) Ltd, Croydon, CR0 4YY

CONTENTS

Yesterday's weirdness is tomorrow's reason why.

Hunter S. Thompson

ACKNOWLEDGEMENTS

Thanks to my editor Hollie for all her hard work; to my agent Humfrey for his very tall wisdom; to Alan for dinners, drinks and meaty tips and most of all, to Dawn, without whom none of this would have been possible.

INTRODUCTION: CAN YOU SEE THE REAL ME, DOCTOR?

I unwrapped a thick cut of grass-fed, organically reared fillet of beef, seasoned it, put it into a hot pan and fried it in a mixture of organic butter and olive oil for three minutes on each side. As the kitchen filled with the smell of caramelised meat my digestive juices ached for the coming feast.

I let it rest for five minutes and then cut into it. It was perfectly medium rare. Rich, tender and intensely savoury, I relished the juicy meat and the delicious, elemental combination of fat and blood.

It was mind-blowingly flavourful; a complete meal in itself that seemed to occupy all my taste buds and senses.

Just two weeks ago this would have been the least likely thing I might have done because two weeks ago I was still a vegetarian. I'd been a vegetarian for twenty-six years. I liked being a vegetarian. It was, quite literally, who I was. For most of those years I'd actually been a vegan, eschewing all animal-derived foods. Oh yeah, that's right. One of *those*.

Don't worry, this isn't a book about vegetarianism. No dreadlocks or earnest lectures about animal rights here. Sod that. There are more important issues to consider, more specifically what is and isn't healthy eating, and how we got to this twenty-first century state of paranoia over what's best to put into our meat-hole. The thing is, I wasn't just a non-meat eater, I was Mr Wholefood: brown rice, healthy vegetable oils, lentils, beans, tofu, nuts, fruit and vegetables. All the stuff the doctors now tell you to eat, well, I started hoovering that all up way back in the mid 1980s when it had only just become part of the 'healthy' eating advice and when very few outside of the small community of hairy, bearded, dope-smoking, wholefood-eating New-Agers had even heard of it.

So for twenty-six years I ate no cholesterol, no animal fats and ate polyunsaturated and wholegrain everything. Go to your local surgery and hand over my food diary and they'd give you a gold star. Your medical man or woman with the stethoscope and that nodding-without-really-listening, slightly condescending attitude, has been advising everyone to base their diet on starchy foods, eat a lot less saturated fat, a lot less animal fat, a lot less cholesterol, a lot less sugar and a lot less red meat for years. It's virtually a religion now.

Look at the Eat Well plate on the NHS website and you'll see the official propaganda all based around these basic principles.

I really was a walking advert for healthy eating. You couldn't eat more of the good stuff and less of the bad stuff than me. If there was a competition for healthy eating, I'd have won hands down – and I was told as much by doctors and nutritionists year after year.

All well and good, but there was trouble in paradise. I was ill. Really ill. And I'd been ill for the majority of those twenty-six years.

For years I had lived with what would come to be known as IBS: Irritable Bowel Syndrome. Starting back in 1993 as a vague feeling of digestive discomfort, it escalated to the point where every meal would leave me feeling like I had lead weights in my gut, my belly bloated and distended and my digestive tract in revolt in the most dramatic and unpleasant way. If you had a cruel sense of humour, you could say I was a dirty protest waiting to happen.

I'd test the sewage system's capacity by passing out vast slurries of burning effluent which left me feeling sweaty and exhausted. This would happen up to seven or eight times a day during the worst period. It was like this to a greater or lesser degree after every meal, every day, every month, every year, on and on and on for seventeen years. Yeah, how d'ya like me now?

What's more, slowly but surely, year after year, I kept putting weight on until I was clinically obese. I peaked in 2008 at fourteen and a half stone, which, for a 5 foot 10 inch tall, medium-build lad, is a lot of blubber to wear. Not big enough to make a freak show but big enough to be very unhealthy. I waddled around, sweating and short of breath when required to do anything slightly physical. I had always been an active sort of bloke. Not exactly sporty – I'm hardly the alpha male type who relishes that kind of masculine bonding. My idea of fun is not holding another man's scrotum in a rugby scrum under the pretence it is a sport. Nonetheless, I was a frequent hiker, walker and swimmer, or at least I had been until the weight began to wrap its fatty tentacles around me.

The bad news didn't stop at being fat. By the time I was forty, I had very, very high cholesterol: a Christ-that-will-kill-you-early reading of 9.2. As my dad had keeled over with a heart attack aged sixty-five, I was put on the new statin drug Atorvastatin. Forty milligrams a day for the rest of my life. Welcome to decrepitude, Johnny. Because it wasn't just the IBS and the sky-high cholesterol; in many other ways I was slowly falling apart. The healthy eating thing wasn't working out well at all. I was suffering from chronic acid reflux; I was always tired and needed to take half an hour naps every afternoon. I suffered from headaches almost every day. I ate paracetamol and Rennies like they were sweets and, oh yeah, my eyesight was failing as well.

Jesus Christ, I thought, how the feck did this happen? It wasn't as if I was an old bloke. I had the low sugar, low-fat, high-fibre, carb-rich, wholegrain, vegetable-based diet that all the health advice had recommended with increasing fervour over the years. I should have been healthy, shouldn't I? Yes, I bloody well should have been but the fact was I had started to fall apart in my early thirties and by my mid forties I was, what the medical establishment would call, totally knackered, son.

And then, suddenly, it all changed when I stuffed my face with some good old fashioned meaty, beaty, big and bouncy products of slaughter, dripping in blood. Bye bye Mr Soya, hello dead sentient creatures.

Twenty-four hours after eating meat all my IBS symptoms had gone! Bloody hell. What was this new voodoo? Had eating animal flesh lifted some sort of hex that had been put on me?

As I began eating meat, I stopped eating high-load carbohydrates such as potatoes and wheat. I cut out all vegetable oils except olive, ate lots of lard, beef dripping, butter, cream and full-fat milk. I ate the fat on chops, the fat on meat, chicken skin, crackling on pork; I ate red meat four or five times a week. Basically I ate a lot of everything that we're told not to eat at all, or only in strict moderation.

In some aspects, it was a diet that my grandparents, born at the end of the nineteenth century, would have known was nutritious and healthy, not because they had been told so by their doctors, by New-Age diet gurus, by freaky-looking people in white coats on the telly or by any other hysterical media outlet, but because they knew previous generations had thrived on it and that they thrived on it themselves.

Today a diet full of saturated fat, red meat, cream and full-fat milk is considered to be a heart attack waiting to happen. Does that come with a defibrillator? Ha ha bloody ha. It is not recommended at all, indeed, my and your doctors will tell you not to indulge in that type of diet. I've been amazed and disgusted. I've wanted to scream in their faces, 'Can you see the real me, doctor?' Partly because I love The Who but mainly because when it came to medical attention, I ran into a brick wall for seventeen years. They had no solutions to my ill health but they still tell me my solution is wrong. This simple and 100 per cent effective remedy was not in any way what the doctor ordered, indeed, the doctor hadn't ordered anything. The doctor hadn't had a bloody clue what to do about it and had pretty much given up. Well done. Thank you and good night. Well, bollocks to them and their idiot ideas because the effect of this new, old-fashioned diet was virtually instant and amazing.

After suffering for seventeen years I could scarcely believe it. But the good news didn't stop there. As the weeks and months progressed, I began to physically change. I got leaner, dropped a lot of body fat and became stronger and fitter. Every aspect of my health and well-being was changed for the better. I felt amazingly energised. It was as though I was suddenly a much younger man.

This was great and weird all at the same time. You get used to how you feel. You don't expect it to change, not for the better anyway. We all seem to be conditioned to believe that life is a journey of slow and inevitable decline until you keel over into your grave, a beaten and exhausted crust of the man you used to be.

But it wasn't just a physical change. For no accountable reason other than the change of diet, I found myself more relaxed and unstressed, despite running my own business in the teeth of a difficult recession and an unrelenting work-load. I was more able to deal with everything; more emotionally even and calm. I even coped with the usually stressful business of finding and moving to a new home.

And it didn't stop there. I developed an increased mental sharpness. Names that had escaped me previously came to mind immediately, I pulled words out of my vocabulary with ease. All aspects of my mental acuity were improved. During the initial period, I finished the final draft of, and published, my first book, *We Ate All the Pies: How Football Swallowed Britain Whole*, which went on to be long-listed for the prestigious William Hill Sports Book of the Year 2010 award.

This was not mere coincidence; I was simply better at everything I did. For years I had been one of those forgetful people in their forties and I put it down to old age. In fact I had put a lot of the degeneration in my physicality down to increasing age: blurry eyesight, the pain in my knees, the stiff joints when getting out of bed, the buzzing headaches, the mid-afternoon weariness – I wrote it all off as due to my age or maybe due to a skinful the night before. I thought it was just how things were; this was what getting older was like. I was wrong. This is what getting older was like on this 'healthy' diet.

But get this: I have now actually stopped wearing glasses for reading because my eyesight improved so much when I changed my diet. Headaches have gone away, never to return – I've not had a single headache in twenty months. Even my libido has increased exponentially. I suddenly started to become aware of a priapic rush of blood, apropos of nothing, the way I did when I was eighteen. It literally felt like being young again, like coming back to life. What the hell was going on?

I was bloody furious with myself for sticking to a diet that made me ill, and with the medical authorities for their years of ineptitude and inability to help when a simple dietary change was all that was needed. I began to wonder how and why the healthy eating advice had become so dogmatic and had been pushed down our throats so often for so long.

So on behalf of every other poor sod who has been crucified with one affliction or another on the cross of this modern dystopian dietary vision of healthy eating, I wanted to get to the truth about food and diet. Since I am thriving in every possible way on a diet I am told isn't healthy for me, it seems to me that at the very least this one-size-fits-all, healthy eating advice is simply inappropriate for some (or many) of us and that this could well be the reason there are so many health issues around food and diet in the twenty-first century, when thirty or more years ago there simply were not.

At a time of healthy eating information overload, at a time of unprecedented availability of food, we are nonetheless utterly messed up when it comes to how and what to eat. So many people are on a diet, off a diet, wondering about a diet, trying to lose weight, trying to stop bloating, indigestion, acid reflux, trying to get more energy, sleep better or just walk up the street without getting out of breath. Throw in feelings of guilt and paranoia and you've got a cauldron of what I like to call fuckedupiness.

This is no way to live, is it? It's bloody insane. A couple of generations ago we worried about having enough food, now we worry about eating too much. It's not a good journey to have made.

I'm not some sort of food guru, I don't wear a white coat, I won't be asking you to shit in a jar so I can tell what's wrong with you and I'm sure as hell not a doctor. I'm just a guy who always wanted to do the right thing – the right thing for me, the right thing for everyone and everything else. The right thing for the planet, even. Ironically, although I never wanted to hurt anyone or anything, I ended up hurting myself badly, day after day.

We may not realise it but our diets have radically changed in the last thirty years and so has our health. It's glaringly obvious that things have gone badly wrong. The stats on things such as Type 2 diabetes, obesity, food intolerances, allergies and many other degenerative diseases show that we are getting fatter and more ill – both physically and mentally.

Could these healthy eating guidelines, and the diet and lifestyle it encourages us to follow, be the main cause of all the problems? Someone in power should be asking this question but the taboos around health on such issues as saturated fat, five fruit and veg a day and too much red meat have become an orthodoxy that no one wants to challenge. Well I'm an ornery sod and that's why I'm here.

We stand on the verge of the next generation living shorter, less healthy, less content lives than the previous one and it has happened on the watch of what we might call the 'healthy eating brigade'. Worse still, despite increased wealth, our well-being appears to have deteriorated too, by which I mean our sense of contentment and happiness with our physical and mental condition. We are eating healthier and getting more unhappy and more ill in ways we never used to get ill. But regardless of this our individual needs have been ignored for this one-size-fits-all notion of healthy living. It is my contention that this advice is simply inap-propriate for many people; indeed, it is making people ill. It helped make me ill. It is also my view that much of what passes for healthy eating advice is little more than supposition, equivocal research and twisted interpretation.

Had I continued to believe the healthy eating propaganda I would still be very ill, so I hope the story I'm about to tell helps shed light on your own situation and perhaps inspires you to think differently about what you feed yourself, and makes you look at how you arrived at the food choices that you make every day.

This book is about how you can get stuck in a rut with your attitude to what you eat. It's about how we've been taken away from a down-to-earth, sensible, sane view of what is wholesome food and replaced it with a hysterical, paranoid, downright sick attitude – a sick attitude which the medical and governmental establishment have colluded on and continue to encourage with a mixture of rigid dogma, ignorance and guesswork, all the while under the influence of vested interest lobbying.

The Meat Fix isn't a pompous lifestyle or diet book written by some weirdo who doesn't live in the real world or some sod who wears bleedin' leg warmers and a leotard. Trust me, I look rubbish in a leotard. I'm damned if I'm going to just sit back and accept what has happened to me. For so long I was just killing myself to live. But not anymore.

considered to be healthy eating, nor was I even curious as to what it might or might not be. We were not so paranoid about it back in the 1970s and early 1980s. Life was tougher. People were on strike all the time, there were power cuts, red vinyl 7-inch singles, punk rock and brightly coloured leg warmers to distract people from worrying about such matters. People who did fret about healthy eating were thought of as fussy. Very few people were fat, so no one thought food was a problem, unless you couldn't get enough, or if the chip shop ran out of battered sausages on a Friday night in which case we got very, very annoyed and would threaten to abuse the greasy, lank-haired chip shop workers with a bottle of non-brewed condiment until they put some more in the fryer.

I'm a 1960s kid, born in 1961, brought up in Hull in East Yorkshire until I was eight and then on Teesside until 1979, when I left home. I had modestly socially aspirant, Tory-voting, working-class parents who had been born into what we would now consider to be grinding poverty in Hull in the 1920s and 1930s, sleeping three or four kids to a bed in back-to-back terraced houses. They spent their childhood huddled around a cup of hot gravel and were grateful for it, and then, just when they'd grown up, the Luftwaffe began bombing them. There was no career advice, no bloody gap year, no finding yourself backpacking around Thailand. They went to work aged fourteen. No choice, no nowt. Bring some money in, kid, and when you're done, could you just nip over the Channel and give Adolf a right kicking, there's a good chap.

As children in the 1960s, my older brother Keith and I inherited a diet from our parents that had changed little since those childhood days. We had a bit more to eat in quantity than they did as children of the depression, and perhaps a little more variety, but what we did eat was very traditional, very basic and repetitive. So repetitive that we had the same meals on the same days of each week for years and years. If it's Monday it must be rissoles in onion gravy. Tuesday was sausage and mash; Wednesday, mince or stew. Thursday, lamb chops or liver. Friday, shepherd's pie, Saturday, fish and chips; Sunday, roast beef or chicken. Week after week, year after year, probably just as my mother's mother had done since the turn of the century.

Compared to the cornucopia of foods available to us today, we had very little deviation from these basics. Of course, as kids we just accepted this state of affairs as normal; this was the way of life for many people like us at the time. Nothing unusual.

Portions were small but we always had three square meals a day. I never left the table hungry but rarely did I leave it full. From an early age, virtually my only stated ambition in life was to have more chips on my plate. I was certain that once I had become a man, I would pile my plate so damn high with fried potatoes that I wouldn't be able to see over the top of them if I climbed a ladder while wearing stilts. This seemed to be as much as anyone could want out of life.

Similarly we were limited to one slice of cake, two biscuits or a single scone at a meal. When fruit was bought we were not allowed to eat it right away. It had to last the week. 'Don't go eating that,' Mam would say as she put a couple of apples and oranges into the fruit bowl. Frugality was a way of life; overeating almost an impossibility.

At Christmas, after a relatively big feast, my tummy actually hurt and it never hurt at any other time of year. It was a Christmas-only experience. This food poverty wasn't because we were the poorest of families or the most frugal; it was just how it was for most people. Food was relatively more expensive and there was no money to load the cupboards until they groaned under the weight.

Before going to school our breakfast was almost always eggs and bacon and fried bread. Dinner was meat with potatoes and two vegetables, tea was something with chips. Supper was cereal or toast. This went on for eighteen long, long years. To say it was a conservative food upbringing would be an understatement but the food regime was pretty spartan, especially when we were young.

Again, in contrast to today, by and large we ate fresh vegetables that were in season because, sensibly, no one thought of importing green beans from Kenya or kumquats from Upper Volta, or wherever. We had root crops, leafy greens and potatoes and, later, frozen peas. That was it, apart from tins of veg such as carrots, peas and, weirdly, mushrooms. Why does anyone buy tinned button mushrooms? They're like mini-testicles in a tin. Not that I know what tiny tinned bollocks look like. Does anyone?

Tomatoes were also canned and only served with a fry up at breakfast. Fresh tomatoes were a summer salad luxury as were any fruit other than apples and pears. Yeah, yeah I know this sounds like a story of grinding poverty but it really isn't. It's just how life was for most of us. Such hairy wonders as kiwi fruit or the dimpled leatheriness of passion fruits were not just not an option, they were unheard of and would most certainly have looked to us like an alien fruit that would have grown on a polystyrene tree on one of those dodgy sets in the original *Star Trek*.

It wasn't just that a wide variety of foodstuffs were not available, it was also very much the case that any kind of alternative diet or regime to our day-to-day food world of brown and beige misery was simply not considered. While some of the more bohemian elements of society might have flirted with eastern-inspired vegetarian ways after smoking dope at university and while there were books suggesting you might want to eat a diet based on cabbages or egg whites or deep-fried socks, these simply had no common currency among the working and lower-middle classes of my youth. Rather, they were considered (if considered at all) as part of a lunatic fringe who had, as my gran would have put it, 'gone all weird on those drug things'. Perhaps subconsciously I absorbed this notion and resolved to give it a try when I got older and had also got all weird on those drug things too. It was the nearest I've ever got to a career.

I realise this sounds like I'm talking about the 1860s not the 1960s, but that just shows how massively food culture and food expectations have altered in the last fifty years for most of us and also how much more wealthy society as a whole is, at least when measured by the amount of stuff bought.

Unlike today, until the early 1970s we ate relatively little heavily processed food and what processed food we did eat had existed since before the First World War, such as Spam, chopped ham, baked beans, digestive biscuits, corn flakes, tins of Heinz tomato soup and Carnation Evaporated Milk. These were virtually the only 'pre-made' food we had apart from bread, which was always Mother's Pride, a weird, sticky-white bread that you could roll up into balls and flick at each other. It was an industrially produced product that was bleached bright white and had such little nutrition in it that by law it had to have various vitamins added to it. Those laws remain in place today. We didn't question the point of eating something so lacking in goodness that it had to have stuff added to it in order to make it nutritious. I don't think many people do, not even now.

All our food as kids was cooked from scratch. There were no TV dinners or pre-prepared meals to heat up and, indeed, had there been so, many housewives (because 'real' 1970s men didn't cook) would have considered it cheating to use them – indeed my gran thought that only a lazy and neglectful mother would have anything to do with modern convenience foods such as frozen fish fingers. She was hard-line about such matters. You made your own food, you knitted your own jumpers, hats and socks. Buying them was a cop out, a cheat, a dereliction of duty. She saw this in the same way we might see having 250 pairs of shoes to choose from today as an excess of consumption and self-indulgence gone wild. I grew up thinking this was mad. Today, I totally understand it.

Like almost all people of their class and generation, my parents, like theirs before them, all thought the traditional English diet was wholesome and that, by contrast, foreign food was 'muck'. Quite sure of this, they based this idea on very little actual knowledge or experience but a lot of bigotry and conjecture.

If there is one word to sum up my childhood food it would be bland. Bland food was trusted by my parents, spicy or strong tasting food was, by contrast, for untrustworthy foreigners and thus to be worried about. This conservative attitude was rife in society at the time, at least among the working class anyway.

Garlic, despite being as British as roast beef, was despised and utterly rejected as an unwanted foreign interloper. Whenever it cropped up on a cookery TV programme, they would sneer with undisguised contempt as though the chef was recommending using dog piss for gravy. They considered garlic to be French – whom they still despised for their poor effort in resisting the Nazis twenty-five years earlier. Yes, they really did. Everyone did. Forgive and forget? You must be bloody joking. Again, this was commonplace. When relations would come around, the thick-armed, big-bosomed Yorkshire or Teesside matriarch of every family would sneer at the TV as a young Delia Smith made garlic mayonnaise. 'Not that bloody garlic stuff again! It makes me feel sick,' they would say with a potent mixture of Yorkshire disgust and maternal indignation.

They all also associated garlic with Indian cooking and they hated that. They looked upon the Indian restaurants, which had begun to spring up even in Teesside by the early 1970s, with disdain even while a younger generation started to embrace them, loading up on hot curry as part of a night on the drink. It wasn't society's finest hour as the poor sods whose lot it was to serve gangs of pissed northerners were often treated with a mixture of racism and curiosity, like some exotic exhibit.

Whichever part of the Asian sub-continent the cuisine actually hailed from, it was always, always labelled by my parents and their ilk as 'that muck' and usually muck made with locally sourced dead cats (the dogs were the preserve of the Chinese, of course). The smell of curry cooking was not something to get you salivating; it was the odour of the unclean and was frightening to them, especially my mother. I think she saw it, in some vein, as a threat to her way of life.

They had a national, if not a racial, stereotype for every citizen of the world and it was to these sensibilities that much of 1970s situation comedy was aimed. The Chinese and Japanese were cruel; the Italians cowardly; hating the Germans was a given even without mentioning the evil-smelling sauerkraut; Scandinavians ate unpleasant fish, spent too much time in saunas ('What's wrong with a good wash?') and had loose morals, especially au pairs. No one had ever met or even seen an au pair, or even knew quite what an au pair did, but somehow, by some sort of sexual osmosis, you knew they were all shaggers.

Americans and Australians were crude, pig-ignorant and ill-mannered. Spanish and Portuguese lazy and possibly criminal. Anyone from the Asian subcontinent was lumped together as unclean and prone to eating their pets; anyone from anywhere in Africa was lazy and still uncivilised unless the British had occupied their country, in which case they were ungrateful for the improvements we had brought; of course the whole of the Middle East was full of dangerous lunatics who had been driven mad from eating hot, garlicky and spicy food. I am not exaggerating; this was drip-fed to me as a kid. Only South America escaped this national and racial stereotyping. For some reason they couldn't come up with anything bad to say about people from places such as Chile, Bolivia or Brazil, nor anything good come to that. Mind, they did like that pan pipe muzak that became popular in the late 1970s. This was about as culturally progressive as life got.

Now, you might think this meant they were all card-carrying fascists but that's not true at all really. They were certainly racist by modern standards but wouldn't have dreamed of being anything other than very polite and civil to anyone they met from another country or race, and they would never have anything to do with the type of people who gravitated toward the emerging National Front movement. They would have been far too strident and rough for them. My mam especially would have seen them as 'common' and far too like the people they'd grown up around and had wanted to climb the social ladder to escape. It was never political, it was always cultural. But nonetheless, it stopped them stepping outside of their prescribed cultural boundaries when it came to food or anything else for that matter.

They didn't hate foreigners really, they were just insecure and frightened of the different cultures they brought with them, which isn't surprising when you consider their background. I'm sure most people of the world who have known little outside of their own culture would be defensive when people from elsewhere move in around them, and there is no more central element to any culture than its food. People get defensive about it, no matter where they're from. Try telling an Italian that pasta lacks nutrition and makes you fat. They don't like it and may try to insert a large bottle of olive oil into you.

It might seem bizarre to think something as common-place as pizza was actually a distant, exotic, foreign food to us but it was. I didn't have my first pizza until the mid 1980s, by which time I was a college-educated kid with a degree in English and History. Yeah, how sophisticated was I? I was more familiar with Pizzaro, Pirandello and PFM than I was with pizza and pasta.

Our only exposure to pasta was via tins of Heinz spaghetti. How bizarre is having spaghetti on toast – a staple meal in the 1970s – being essentially wheat served on wheat? It's like having a sandwich and putting bread in as the filling! This has always bothered me.

As soon as more fancy processed food arrived on the shelves in the mid 1970s, we lapped it up at the first opportunity, hoovering down all manner of powdered, dried, frozen, weird plastic stuff. Such things as a Vesta Chow Mein were more like a by-product of the chemical industry and looked and tasted like that too. But luckily, growing up on Teesside in the shadow of the chemical industry gives you a taste for such things and I craved them, probably because they were loaded with monosodium glutamate and, for all I know, nuclear waste material from Sellafield, then called good old-fashioned Windscale.

Like all kids of that generation, we were incredibly active the whole time, possibly because we consumed vast amounts of sugar. It was non-stop. Sugar on cereal, in tea, in cakes and buns and biscuits at every meal, in the never ending river of jam served on bread for tea and from the local sweet shop in the form of all manner of irresistible cheap sweets.

I bloody loved cheap sweets and consequently I was an excitable, some might say damn annoying child, frequently running around the walls, making odd screeching sounds and constantly prattling away in a stream of noises and made-up words. I always was a bit manic and very, very excitable. This was put down to just being my nature but was actually almost certainly due to the sugar and the colourings that sweets and pop were dyed to make them bright colours. I recall Cresta, a strange can of pop, advertised by a very cool polar bear who told us, 'It's frothy, man.' Indeed it was. Then again so was the local river and that was because of the concoction of efflu-ent and chemicals that was pumped directly into it. There were parallels. Cresta was odd. The green one was lime, red strawberry, purple blackcurrant, but all tasted vaguely simi-lar and yet indescribable, like nothing that had ever existed in nature. It was sweet but kind of bitter and left you a little nauseous and with a sore throat afterwards. In no universe other than 1970s Britain could this be construed as a good thing; soft drinks should not agitate your tonsils and leave you feeling as though you've been maced by the riot police, but we knocked the stuff back all summer long.

I think after a childhood of beige foods, the brilliant colours of the mid and late 1970s artificial food and drink were bound to be appealing because you've got to remember that for all that the 1960s are swinging in the history books, in Hull and on Teesside they were not. For most of this period, life really was much more like the pre-war make-do-and-mend world than a temple to far-out and groovy 1960s coolness. The only acid in our life was acetic – vinegar. On chips. Malt, of course. We'd never heard of cider vinegar. Like garlic and bread, cider and vinegar were two words that simply didn't belong together. A trip meant a day out in Darlington, not a psychedelic union with the godhead, not unless he or she was visiting Darlington at the time, anyway.

Our house was a temple to thrift. Mam would keep drawers full of small bits of string and sheets of brown paper, ironed paper bags, wax paper, drawing pins, small pots of glue, paper clips and brown rubber bands – all kept 'just in case'. Just in case of what? Who knows? It was a way of life; a kind of mantra to the infinite possibilities of existence which might, just might, mean that in nine years' time the brown paper bag you had ironed, yes ironed, and put away, might be needed. It was like a protection against the uncertain tides of life. If you had enough odd bits of string, knicker elastic, bottle tops or rubber washers in a drawer, then you could cope with whatever surprises life had in store right up to, but not including, nuclear war.

Nothing was ever thrown out. The idea of throwing away, say, a jam jar, would have been laughed at because a clean, used jam jar had a whole lifetime of work ahead of it in our house from holding turps, pens, tadpoles, flour, paint or being filled with petrol and used as a bomb if rioting broke out.

You didn't throw away a resource like that! Old shirts were torn up and used as dusters, old trousers put away for use in the garden until they were threadbare at which point they were filled with newspaper and sacrificed like some modern-day Wicker Man on the 5 November bonfire going down in a blaze of glory after a lifetime of use.

If we'd just had a bonfire, when clothes finally became unwearable and exhausted we would give them to the rag-and-bone man who would come around with a cart each week. In return we'd get a balloon and consider this rather fantastic. It's funny how, when your expectations are low, such small things can seem so exciting.

In hindsight this all sounds very worthy – an early form of downsizing perhaps – but the truth was we just had sod all, even though we can't have been the worst off family because my dad, controversially, was the first in his family to get a white collar job working for British Rail, which was seen as rampant social climbing and by the more left wing in our ranks as a rejection of his roots, which indeed it was. As those roots were little more than living in a hole in the ground huddled under a tarpaulin, it was perfectly understandable.

So my food culture was inevitably set in these relatively spartan years. This was what I thought food was. For all I knew, everyone else in the UK ate like this too. We were not exposed to any other way of life at all. We had no notion at all about what was healthy and what was not.

The meat we ate was usually mince, cheap cuts and the organ meats about which we were not squeamish in the slightest; indeed, liver and onions was one of the few very tasty meals we had.

We rarely ate fish except from the chip shop and the occasional tin of salmon (only for Sunday tea), tuna and pilchards. We also rarely ate pork or gammon. There was nothing exotic like venison, duck or game nor any sort of steak. That was only for eating in a Berni Inn, never at home.

The Berni Inn was a very 1970s institution, even though they survived until the mid 1990s. Ours in Stockton was at the top of the High Street and was generally considered to be a 'smoothie' pub. This just meant that the punters didn't wear jeans, favouring the large billowing, three button high-waisted Oxford bags that were so popular in the mid 1970s. And they went to discos too. And danced. This was not rock 'n' roll.

It was supposed to be more classy than your average boozer. This view was based on the fact it was open-plan and had fitted carpets throughout which, at least in the north, was thought of as posh, modern interior design. This was because most pubs were typically either a couple of small, smoky, grubby rooms or one cavernous, brightly lit, plaster-walled altar to drinking. Only the lounge of a pub was carpeted and, as a man, you only used it on Sunday afternoons or when trying to impress a future father-in-law with your sophisticated, monied ways because beer was often a penny or two more expensive in the lounge. You didn't get a carpet and a few horse brasses for nowt y'knaw! So the Berni seemed lush and decadent by comparison. Some older, hardline geezers considered it far too lavish and thus an insult to your northern masculinity. Too much comfort and soft furnishings was, well, homo-bloody-sexual.

There were frequent fights inside and outside the Berni because, for some reason, the smoothies were always keen on punching each other after ten pints of Harp lager. One night, as a young under-age drinker, hoping to appear older and more sophisticated, my friend and I went in. But what to drink in this red, orange and brown plastic paradise? We usually supped the local bitter, Cameron's Strongarm, but we were now in The Berni; surely we should be drinking something more classy. We looked at the menu on the side of the bar and there at the bottom it said 'Angostura Bitters 10p'. Blimey, we thought, that's a cheap pint and it must be a foreign beer. Imported. Very classy. We'll have two pints of that.

'Er ... two pints of Angostura Bitters please mate,' I said with as much confidence as a 16-year-old boy who looks twelve years old could muster. To our horror the bloke behind the bar roared out in laughter. 'George, George, come here,' he called to his co-worker, 'these lads want a pint of Angostura Bitters, shall we give it to them?' George also roared with laughter. We were by now puce with embarrassment though we didn't know why.

The barman put a bottle on the bar counter in front of us, 'That's your Angostura Bitters son, it's to go in cocktails you daft lad. Now, pint of Harp is it?'

Well, how were we to know? Anyway, as well as being a pub for men with well-trimmed sideburns and 36-inch flared trousers to drink in, it was also a restaurant.

That being said, it wasn't a proper restaurant really and that was exactly why it was so very popular with the working and lower middle classes. More accurately it was a pub that did food. This might seem unexceptional now but back in the 1970s it was a brilliant, stellar new concept.

It offered the chance for a meal out but without any of the intimidation a meal at a proper restaurant held. There'd be no wine waiters or French menus listing foods you'd never heard of. No worrying about which was the fish knife and whether it was OK to ask for tomato sauce. And you could drink pints of beer with your dinner.

All of these worries, in common with many millions from their background, kept my parents away from restaurants pretty much for their whole lives. The exception they made was for the Berni. Admittedly, this was only used once every couple of years but if a meal out was necessary, it would happen in the Berni.

So it was that when I passed my O-Levels, I was taken there as a reward. It wasn't the kind of reward I actually wanted but I didn't want to appear ungrateful.

The Berni menu never changed. It was always a prawn cocktail for starter, steak and chips for your main, and Black Forest gateau for pudding. Now, you have to remember that a prawn cocktail was fabulously upmarket for us. It contained avocado which we simply never saw in the green grocers and it contained prawns which were also, for some reason, thought to be posh. But crucially, it was drenched in a mixture of salad cream and tomato sauce, which was romantically called rose sauce and took away the unfamiliar taste of the avocado and prawns. So your prawn cocktail was simultaneously both posh, modern and yet comfortingly familiar. And you ate it with a spoon. No bloody weird cutlery needed. Excellent.

The steak was a T-bone. The waiter asked my dad how we wanted ours cooked because this was a decision that men made. Who knows why? Like everyone in the 1970s he said 'well done' because the idea that your meat might ooze blood was thought wrong, dirty even. It wasn't cooked properly. It was under-done. But I was so naïve at first I assumed asking for a steak well done meant well cooked, done to a decent standard. It seemed to make sense.

So it arrived burnt, dry and tough and you expected it to be like that. However, if it was slightly less burnt, dry and tough than the meat you usually ate at home, which it was, then it still seemed as though you were living high on the hog. And it came with chips, so it all seemed like a slightly better version of 'normal' food.

The cake you had for pudding was usually smothered in some sort of synthetic cream out of a can. Out of a can! Very posh. Any fool could pour some simple, honest cream; you had to be a genius to get it in a can under high pressure so it squirted out. This was progress. It felt like you were eating in the space age. The Berni menu was considered the best of all worlds: familiar but slightly more posh than home-cooked food.

However, as good as the food was, eating out with your parents when neither you nor they are used to eating out was a tense, fraught occasion. While the Berni Inn setting reduced the chances for some social faux pas involving obscure vegetables or unfamiliar cutlery, you were still in public and thus couldn't drop food down your shirt, chew with your mouth open or belch loudly. This was a considerable inhibition. Plus the pressure to talk was also almost unbearable. I always felt as though you were supposed to look like you were having a good time and were a happy family, so you'd sit there sweating bullets, manically trying to think of something to say and not get into an argument.

There was a palpable sense of relief when it was all done, the bill paid and we could walk out of the door. Going home was definitely the best bit of going out to eat.

Given our relatively frugal menu as kids it's no surprise that, like almost all kids at the time, I grew up without an ounce of fat on me despite eating an undoubtedly high-fat diet. Even starting an early drinking career aged fifteen and a half didn't seem to put much weight on me.

In hindsight, this really interests me. In the 1960s and 1970s, in my experience, almost no one ate a low-fat diet in the working or lower-middle classes. In fact, the working class who were short of money and food, actively sought out fat for nutrition. We ate suet puddings every week, we ate the fat on our chops because almost all the chop was fat. We ate fish and chips deep-fried in lard, or better still, beef dripping. Our bacon and eggs were also fried in lard. Indeed, we ate something home-made called Lardy Cake which was a basic cake often presented with custard on. Milk was full fat. I'm not sure if skimmed milk even existed in the 1960s. We ate full fat cheese – only cheddar cheese of course – or occasionally in moments of high adventure, some Cheshire. And we ate eggs every day.

So by modern standards we ate a very high-fat diet, no doubt about it – and it was a high-saturated-fat diet – but neither of us kids were anything other than skinny and so were the vast majority of adults. We also ate tonnes of sugar but our bodies didn't lay it down as fat the way it seems to on kids today. A high-fat diet didn't make us fat, contrary to what we might be told today about such things. This wasn't just me, it was 98 per cent of kids from all social classes. The chubster was a very rare exception and, consequently, somewhat picked upon by the nastier children, presumably driven to such rage by a cocktail of food additives, sugar and sniffing their mother's lighter fuel. Or was that just me? It's not that everyone was emaciated, you sometimes saw chunkier older women and older blokes with a beer gut but they were in far less numbers than today. People in their twenties, thirties and forties were almost never fat. It was a genuinely rare condition.

I would have loved to sit in front of a computer for eight hours a day; it would have suited my mentality perfectly to lose myself in some role-playing game in a fictional world. As that wasn't an option I'd disappear with friends all day to what seemed remote parts of Stockton during summer holidays, walking miles and miles and miles. Hard to recall now but cars were much less prevalent, even into the mid 1970s. I rarely got lifts anywhere, instead you walked. If you wanted to go somewhere that was under five or six miles away you always walked unless it was terrible weather and then you'd maybe get the bus. Even at sixteen and seventeen I'd walk three or four miles into town to go drinking. I was on the move the whole time. Indolence was not part of life. It couldn't be. You'd never have done anything otherwise.

So food and lifestyle-wise that was how I arrived at being an adult in 1979, eager to leave home behind. I had little experience or knowledge of food, little cooking skill and a very under-developed palate. Growing up in the north east of England in the 1970s you simply didn't ever meet a vegetarian, nor were you exposed to the whole idea of non-meat eating as a philosophy. I simply don't think it ever crossed anyone's mind to be vegetarian. No one knew a vegetarian, nor had ever heard of one, let alone a vegan. Even Paul McCartney kept it quiet for a while. I certainly wouldn't have ever imagined myself embracing such a lifestyle a few years hence. I'm not even sure I had heard of it as a potential lifestyle. It certainly wasn't the sort of thing a Teesside teenager did, not even a sensitive boy with a fondness for beat poetry and over-amplified guitar solos. If you'd asked anyone about it, they'd have thought it very weird and almost certainly bad for you. What would you eat? Grass?

The main focus of attention was on having enough to eat. No one worried much how it was grown, what it was or even where it came from, which is presumably why I wasn't in the least bit squeamish about dead animals' corpses in the butchers or anywhere else for that matter.

My grandad Fred kept a rusty old water butt full of blood from the slaughterhouse by the back door of his council house in Castleford and it fascinated me from an early age. I recall being very sensible and practical about it. I knew it was animal blood and I knew it was good for his garden, so I didn't recoil from it; rather, it seemed somehow special.

'Show us the blood Fred!' I'd excitedly demand when we went to visit and he'd lift off the old dustbin lid that covered the butt and there underneath was a dark black-purple, thick-looking liquid with an oily skin on top, to which flies had got stuck and drowned.

Does anyone except a serial killer have a barrel of blood in their garden anymore? Is it even legal? Surely there's some sort of health and safety legislation that prevents you having red corpuscles in your garden.

Castleford in West Yorkshire was a mining town. Fred worked down the pit his whole life and had the rattle in his lungs to prove it. Like many miners he grew all his own vegetables in the back garden. He used the blood as a fertiliser, dipping a rusty watering can into the dark viscous liquid, diluting it with some water and pouring it onto seedlings and such. Then he'd scatter ground-up animal bones and rake it into the soil; again these had come from the local slaughterhouse.

He also caught rabbits. I don't know where he caught them in the middle of Castleford but there was often a couple hanging up in the back kitchen. It was much needed free food. Getting things for nothing was an art form the old bugger was very good at, which was just as well because he and my gran had very little money. He'd follow the rag-and-bone man, who pulled a cart with a horse just like *Steptoe and Son* at least into the late 1960s, carrying a zinc bucket and shovel waiting for the horse to open its bowels. In fact the sound of horses' hooves on the road would always send him sprinting to get his bucket because there was competition for horse manure. If he didn't get to it first, someone else would get the golden nuggets. It was perfect for the garden of course and, again, free of charge.

Again, this now sounds like some bucolic, sepia-tinted Victorian scene, but it was commonplace just forty years ago. I say that like forty years is nothing but it's gone by sodding quickly.

It wasn't just through visiting him that I was exposed to bloody matters. Until the mid 1970s at least, everyone bought meat from a butcher because supermarkets were few and far between and the days of sanitised, frozen, boxed or packed-up meat cuts were still some years away. So there was no escaping the reality of butchery. This was a good thing. It meant there was no hiding from the reality. No dressing it up. No pretending it wasn't a corpse. It didn't bother us.

The butchers my mam used in Hull had sawdust on the floor. The odour of the place was a distinctive mixture of pungent pine dust and the rich-scented animal blood. There hanging on the wall were the carcasses of pigs, massive shoulders of beef, chickens hanging by their legs and occasionally a pheasant or rabbit. They would cut you a piece of the animal of your choice right there and then. There was no messing around, no being sensitive to vegetarians or small children's delicate sensibilities or to the squeamish meat eater. It was wrapped in newspaper and you took it home, the blood sometimes soaking through the waxed paper it was put in before being wrapped in the *Hull Mail* or the *Evening Gazette*. We accepted it as a normal way of life and it never upset me nor made me think of being a non-meat eater. Now I wish I never had. I had inherited a perfectly sensible attitude to such matters which had served people very well since the dawn of time.

When I left home for college in Newcastle I really enjoyed shopping for myself and being responsible for my own food. It never once intimidated me, I never missed home, never missed Mam's cooking. Well, who can miss rubbery, overcooked bacon and egg flans?

I was mad keen to be independent, get away from the conservatism of home life and embrace a more bohemian existence that would essentially involve a lot of sex and drugs and rock 'n' roll, though if I could have had the sex and the rock 'n' roll, I was quite prepared to do without the drugs. I'd go food shopping in the Grainger Market, a fantastic old indoor market in the centre of Newcastle which housed lots of butchers along with fruit and veg, sweets, haberdashers, clothes and even an old Marks and Spencer Penny Bazaar dating back to the turn of the century.

The Grainger Market is a Grade I Listed Building, built in 1835 when it was considered to be Europe's finest and most spacious indoor market. By 1979 it was still largely unchanged and was a great place to buy cheap meat, suitable for the student on a budget. This was basic stuff. No corporate branding, no fancy packaging, all the prices were written in felt-tip on wipe clean plastic signs or bits of paper. They were all family businesses and many had been there for several generations.

Again, this was naked butchery in all its slaughtered glory. Dead animals hanging up everywhere. Still I wasn't persuaded that being vegetarian was a suitable response to all the bloody corpses. It didn't even occur to me because, in common with most people, I was not inquisitive about, had no idea about and received no instruction on what was or wasn't a healthy diet from any medical professional at any point in my first twenty-one years of life. Healthy eating wasn't quite the obsession in popular culture that it is today.

It's also worth remembering that there were no programmes on TV about such matters, no doctors on the sofa of morning TV programmes. There was little in the press about it either or at least not to the extent it is today. There was some broad agreement that smoking was probably bad for you, though many dissented from that view on the basis that if it was so bad how come their grandad had smoked all his life and was ninety-one years old? But the reduction of smoking among the population had been reducing the heart attack rate for the previous fifteen years.

In the absence of formal education on such matters, what to eat was mainly just handed down through the generations.

It certainly wasn't taught to us at school. Indeed, as a male of the species, I was not allowed to even do domestic science at school in case it turned me into a girl or perhaps a raging homosexual. In an incredible piece of 1970s sexism only girls could learn how to cook, though I doubt this included any information on what food was good and what bad. My partner (I hate the word partner but what word can you use after thirty-one unmarried years together?) Dawn tells me her lessons in 'Cookery and Sewing' involved learning about good housekeeping, managing your weekly budget, how to bake a cake and how to perform a good enough blow job to stop your husband abandoning you in favour of the estate bike.

Health in relation to food simply wasn't on the regular person's agenda in that era. The one and only time this was even talked about in our house was one day around the summer of 1975. I was fourteen and was having a Sunday 'run out' in the car to Roseberry Topping, a wonky-shaped hill outside of Teesside that was a popular place for a walk, during which my mam told me that my now fat dad had 'a weak heart' and had been told to lose weight.

I asked how he was going to do that and she said the doctor had told him to cut down on potatoes and bread. It was typical of the repressed emotional nature of my family that this was never ever mentioned again, but the attempted reduction of carbohydrate in his diet must have been a temporary effort because he continued to gain weight and I don't remember his portion of starch being markedly smaller and it was certainly never absent. I don't think this heart condition was necessarily attributed to diet, more it was considered simply 'weak' as though this was an innate physical problem which being overweight would merely aggravate.

Ironically, my dad was lean for most of his life – I look at photos of him in the army during the war and he's all muscle and no fat and in his wedding photos in 1955 he's just the same. In holiday snaps of us in Bournemouth in 1971, he was nearly fifty and just starting to put some fat on his bones. Between the early 1970s and late 1970s this all changed. Suddenly he gained weight, putting on a big belly. This corresponded to an increase in his wages as he moved through the middle-management ranks. He wasn't a drinker at all but he did love eating and he was increasingly office-bound. He was only about five foot six so the weight sat heavy on him.

Significantly, in the 1970s we got slightly more wealthy and food got a little cheaper. I wouldn't really have known we were better off were it not for the new three-piece suite that turned up one day as well as the new colour telly. By today's standard of opulence this was nothing, but in our world of relative impoverishment it was huge. He also got a company car, a mustard-coloured Austin 1100 with freezing in the winter, skin-melting in the summer, plastic seats

With this up-tick in money came an increase in his sugar and carbohydrate consumption as Mam bought more cakes and confectionery instead of home-baking. It also meant we ate far more 'shop-bought' food. She also stopped using lard in the chip pan and used Spry Crisp and Dry from the mid 1970s instead. My gran, her mother, wasn't pleased. She thought vegetable oil was a modern fad. She liked lard and beef dripping and said oil made chips greasy and almost inedible. Mam clearly liked using the oil precisely because of this. She saw it as modern, as moving on.

Dad never did any exercise and now drove everywhere. This all starts to sound like a typical twenty-first century life-style now doesn't it? More processed food, more sugar, more vegetable fat and a day spent behind a desk and a wheel. His physical response was to bloat up quickly. By the late 1970s he had a sizeable belly and had the familiar apple shape so common today.

Obviously, I didn't know it at the time but when I left home in 1979 he was just eight years from death by a massive heart attack aged just sixty-five. Lights out.

It fell to me to go to the old family house where he had lived on his own and clear it out after his death. Now that was spooky. Everything was left as it was when he made his last trip from the kitchen to the settee on which he expired, a settee that still had police sheet and yellow tape across it saying 'Warning: Biohazard'. Yikes.

'What comes out of you when you die?' I asked Dawn who was, thankfully, with me. Being a Geordie and thus made of stern stuff she fearlessly lifted the police covering and peered under.

'Looks like a bit of blood, doesn't smell of anything worse,' she said, bravely sniffing the air. The indentation from where he'd sat at the fatal moment was still evident. Right there and then it made me realise that for most of us that is just about all we leave behind.

We come and we go. Just another life in the fathomless billions of existences that there have been and will be.

We think we're so special, so great, we humans, but that's all we are, an indentation on the cushion of existence. As odd as it might sound, I found that quite comforting and still do. Once you grasp the fact that we are little more than a speck of dust that comes and goes in the blinking of the cosmic eye, then it deflates the hubris and pomposity so innate to our species. Maybe if we could keep that in mind, we'd stop beating the crap out of each other and spend our short lives in more peace and harmony. Or maybe it just isn't in our headbanger monkey DNA to do that.

When I started eating meat again, this experience at the house came back to me very powerfully. I realised that by being a vegetarian I had got away from this essential understanding of our place in the scheme of things and had tried to elevate myself outside of our place as animals in the cycle of life and death as though we were excluded from the wheel of existence somehow. That what I had chosen to do by being a vegetarian was, at core, deeply unnatural, despite the fact that for the whole time I didn't eat meat I would have argued the exact opposite was true.

My mother, though divorced from him for a few years prior to his death, survived him but was never well and hadn't been so since the mid 1970s, though exactly what was wrong was never really discussed. I think it started with what Gran would have called 'downstairs trouble' and developed into mental difficulties.

She remained a committed smoker all her life and in the early 1980s developed severe paranoid schizophrenia for which she eventually received ECT treatment. That seemed to wipe away who she had been and replaced it with a calmer but blanker person. When I began to research my own diet and how it had affected me, I began to wonder just how what my parents had eaten, especially in the mid 1970s to early 1980s, had affected their subsequent medical conditions.

There is no divorcing what we consume from how we are both physically and mentally. Later, in Dawn's worst symptoms of hypothyroidism and depression caused by twenty-six years of soya rich diet, which includes a kind of mental fragility and inability to cope with stress of any kind, I recognised in her some of the same symptoms I saw in the early stages of Mother's mental deterioration. Fortunately Dawn, through twenty-first century research, was able to learn what had happened and begin recovery. Crucially she wasn't reliant on the narrow, flawed view of a single doctor. In the 1970s and 1980s, there were only strong narcs and brain frying electricity, rather tragically.

So there I was in September 1979, newly installed in Newcastle Poly's self-catering halls of residence, on my own at last, with few basic cooking skills. I could fry a few pieces of meat, I could make spaghetti bolognese and I was a dab hand at putting Marmite onto Ryvitas. Of course, away from home for the first time, food takes a back seat to everything else.

A chip shop on Percy Street, dubbed The Hairy Pie, was food central for me. It was run by a hirsute Middle-Eastern gentleman who presumably shed the hairs that clung so tenaciously to the chips and pies. At such times in life, even if it should be, nutrition is not important at all, whereas getting laid and drinking very much is. Even if nutrition had been important I'm not exactly sure where I would have obtained any information about diet from.

It was while at college in my first year that I pulled Dawn. She was the primo rock chick of my year and was among those who counted themselves in the long-haired rock 'n' roll fraternity – quite a sex and drugs and rock 'n' roll style catch. My Geordie mate Tony looked on from afar one night and said to me approvingly, 'There goes young Dawn ... they reckon she gans, like.' And he was right.

Our meeting revolved around Thin Lizzy, who were playing Newcastle City Hall that night. Dawn was going to see them, while I had failed to get tickets and was going to see ex-Thin Lizzy man Brian Robertson's new band, Wild Horses, who were playing the Poly Ballroom. So it was that we met up later that night as Wild Horses bashed out their under-appreciated rock 'n' roll. Standing right in front of us was Thin Lizzy head honcho Phil Lynott, presumably perusing his old guitarist's new work. To try and impress

Dawn I said I'd get her an autograph of the great man of whom she was a big fan. I coolly strode up to Phillo with pen and paper and requested his signature to which he replied, with a degree of Celtic lyricism, 'Fuck off.' I slunk back a beaten man.

But the Nicholson charm is a stain that is hard to wash off, like blood or chip fat perhaps. We've been together for thirty-one years now, never bothering to get married. We could never quite see the point of it. Like Joni said, 'We don't need no piece of paper from city hall.'

Within a couple of years, under the influence of John Seymour's seminal book *The Complete Book of Self-Sufficiency*, we were living in the north of Scotland on the Black Isle. We'd rented a small cottage with a bit of land and were organically growing all our own fruit and veg and generally being hippies, dude. It was like we'd retired aged twenty-two. This was all well before Hugh Fearnley-Whittingstall and his River Cottage trip. He was still at Oxford when we were doing this and of course he had lots of money, or at least the ability to borrow lots of money. Dirty northern toerags like us never had such luxuries. Not that I'm bitter. Much.

This was all well before most people had even heard of producing food organically. Those that had disparagingly called it growing by 'muck and magic' as opposed to growing using delicious, toxic hardcore chemicals. Funny how this and the wholegrain, wholefood outlook that went with it both started out as very left-field, weirdo hippy/green bits of philosophy and became, within twenty years, regular and quite mainstream.

Within a year we had become around 75 per cent self-sufficient during the summer, growing and storing all our own veg and fruit. There wasn't enough land for us to keep animals but we did have six hens that lived in a hen house painted with a rainbow, inevitably. This was actually the converted innards of a twin-wheel transit van, which we had turned into a kind of caravanette while living in Walker in a brief flirtation with being a crusty – not that we called them that at the time, this was just before the crusty movement really started. We ended up selling the van to some gypsies without ever having lived in it, stripping out its contents and recycling the hardboard lining as a hen house. Of course. Who hasn't done that?

Then one day a hen became egg-bound. This happens quite often and the poor lass went downhill fast. She was suffering and the other hens, in a decidedly un-sisterly manner, started picking on her, pecking out her feathers. No amount of exhortation for them to leave her alone worked. They were severely uncool hens, picking on the weak one among them with the gimlet eye of a vicious spinster in an old people's home. We made the decision to wring her neck – it was for the best, she was clearly on the way out and not to do so would make her suffer longer.

This turned out to be tougher to do than we had imagined. Firstly, I was too much of a wuss to do it. Death is a short word but is a big thing to impose on a living creature. I held her under my arm, her quick breaths making her soft, feathery chest rise and fall. She was warm and very obviously alive. Hens are not bright creatures, they have almost no brains and are set up to do a few things: scratch, peck and lay eggs, primarily. As anyone who has seen hens dust-bathing will testify, they are clearly sentient creatures who feel pleasure and pain and, sadly, pain was what I was about to inflict on her.

I was supposed to be trying to follow John Seymour's instructions on how to dispatch a bird. I stood and rehearsed it in my mind. But I just couldn't bring myself to do it. Suddenly having the power of life and death over this lovely living creature seemed too great a burden. Who was I to play God with this bird's life? Then again, she was going to be dead soon enough and destined to die a painful death too, so who was I to let that happen?

Dawn's more robust Geordieness took over and she took her and gave her an almighty yank; pull away from you and twist, that was the manoeuvre. Only for some reason it didn't work. She pulled away and twisted and the neck distended and went floppy but Henny Penny was still very much alive. Oops. Now we had a bird wandering around with a half-broken, floppy neck. I have to say, hens being phlegmatic creatures who seem to quickly accept their lot in life, she seemed remarkably unstressed by this turn of events and tried to peck as usual but as she could no longer support her own head this proved impossible and it just dragged on the floor, which in turn made her unbalanced and fall over. Oh dear. It was funny and yet appalling.

This made us panic. What had we done? Why wouldn't she die? We stared at her hoping she'd miraculously expire. But she didn't. I picked up the axe that I used to chop wooden logs with, reasoning this was as good a way as any of ending things. However, it wasn't very sharp and we both feared a headless chicken running around spouting blood.

So Dawn picked her up again, put her under her arm, gripped the neck firmly and proceeded to yank and wring the poor creature's neck so fiercely and furiously for such a long time that she stripped all the feathers and skin off the neck, pulling and pulling and pulling until the bird was finally lifeless. She gave up life without a sound, as you would if a massive animal was pulling at your neck for five minutes.

What a bloody relief. For a moment I had feared we had an immortal chicken on our hands that would forever haunt us with her long floppy neck.

We then plucked her, gutted her and boiled her. There was nothing on her at all after being ill and even the cat, who loved chicken and indeed any meat of any sort, wouldn't eat her. An inglorious end really.

This whole process was emotionally draining and more than a little upsetting even though, in among the panicking, we couldn't help laugh at the ludicrous nature of it all. If we were like this with a hen what would we be like with a big, intelligent, rebellious and reluctant-to-be-killed mammal like a pig? It really brought home to us what eating meat really meant. Life and death.

We began to seriously doubt that killing our own animals was for us after all.

Suddenly, eating meat began to seem like a massive self-indulgence when there was plenty of other food available. We couldn't kill it ourselves so why should we ask someone else to do the dirty work? So we made what turned out to be a big decision. Not that we thought it was that big at the time. We just thought, quite casually, it'd probably be for the best if we didn't eat meat any more if we couldn't grow and slaughter it ourselves. It seemed a fairly reasonable position. It also seemed logical that if we were not going to eat meat, we should also not eat dairy produce, as the dairy industry was just as much a part of the slaughter industry. So, vegan it is then. Ok, let's bloody well do it.

So on 13 January 1984 we had our last meat, a couple of slices of bacon and drew a line in the sand. No more slaughter. It felt great. It was exciting. A brave new world.

As soon as we had made the decision, we never looked back. It was never a case of 'cheating' or even missing it in any way whatsoever; quite the opposite. It meant that we quickly learned how to cook with a whole host of different and unusual foods that were previously totally alien to us. That was really stimulating, so much so that it felt as though stopping eating meat rather than narrowing our diet had actually liberated us to learn about, and eat, a wide range of new exciting foods such as chickpeas! Yes, chickpeas! Well, you've got to remember that such things were not available in most supermarkets at the time. They were weird and unheard of to all but the wholefood brigade and the middle-class gourmand.

At the same time that we embarked on this lifestyle change, governments from USA to Europe were now recommending that people cut down on eating animal fats, cholesterol and red meat in favour of more starchy foods, fruit and vegetables, and wholegrains. The new healthy eating advice was all over newspapers and magazines. This sounded very much like a hippy, wholefood, almost vegetarian diet. It sounded like our diet. At least it did to our ears.

The whole 'healthy eating' wave was breaking; eating animals wasn't just morally wrong, it was also bad for you. 'Yes!' we thought. Get in! Buy one lifestyle and get another healthy one free. It all made sense and it was modern and fashionable, even.

Once we had established this as a way of life, we really loved it. As a vegan you are top of the moral food tree – or so you think, anyway. You are a big notch above mere vegetarians and the vegetarians know it. So vegans win. No one will admit this but there is no argument. Being vegetarian is really a bit wimpy. Being vegan is hardcore and, at least on one level, morally defensible and consistent. Being a vegetarian is a cop out. You can't on the one hand say you are against the death of animals for food and eat cheese and milk that comes from the dairy industry which kills and has to kill thousands of animals every day.

To the more militant vegan, the vegetarian is little better than the meat eater: someone too weak to give up animal products; too enslaved to the killing machine. Vegans really shouldn't be lumped in with vegetarians because they're often very different in their motivations and principles.

By the end of the 1980s, mainstream food retailers started to embrace the vegetarian pound. You could buy dried vege-burger mixes, made from soya and some unholy flavourings, from most supermarkets. I vividly remember discovering soya milk in the Co-op in Anfield Plain in County Durham, as unpretentious and working class a place as you could find anywhere, and thinking, 'Bloody hell, we're winning.' The mainstream was coming on board.

By the early 1990s, all the healthy eating advice was now unified in emphasising the importance of eating lots of vegetables, polyunsaturated fats and avoiding the evil of cholesterol. Our own view of our diet was one of private but smug righteousness. This takes me some courage to admit today because who really wants to confess to being a smug bastard? But we were because it had all swung our way. We were doing it right.

Meat seemed even more like yesterday's thing than it had in 1984; an old-fashioned notion, clung to by those who were simply out of touch with the new thinking. By the late 1980s, surveys were coming out saying that at least half of the population of the UK were trying to cut down their red meat intake. In the five years since we'd quit meat, this seemed a huge 'advance'. The salmonella in eggs issue and the scandal of BSE only further endorsed our choice.

In the early 1990s we fled these shores for the sunshine and sea of California, living in Laguna Beach, right on the beach. We'd had a few trips to the west coast and loved the sun, sea, sand and classic rock lifestyle. It appealed to our old hippy instincts to some degree but it was also far more progressive in its attitude to our eating requirements There was a long existing community of veggie and vegan establishments to whom you didn't have to explain your weird beliefs nor did you have to ask if the chips were fried in lard or vegetable oil. Being vegan was one of the lesser freaky lifestyle choices in fact. People understood. It was also the case that many people in California were hugely concerned about healthy eating, which, de facto, led restaurants to have options we could enjoy. On top of that there was classic rock radio, three hundred days of sunshine a year, cold beers and a swimming pool. Having grown up in the old north of England it felt like we'd died and gone to heaven. Endless date palms arcing up to an infinite blue sky. Teesside it wasn't.

For restless, rootless people like us, to live among other restless, rootless people was as near to having an extended family that either of us had. You felt as though you were among your own people, people who shared your values and outlook on life. Even though it attracted plenty of flaky dippy hippies who were too far out for our working-class northern nature, we still saw this as better and more fun than the old-fashioned meat-heads. I'd sit on the rocks watching the sun melt into the liquid mercury of the Pacific Ocean as some local girl did what she called 'ballet dancing to the music of the ocean' but which to me looked more like a form of random epilepsy. I just fucking loved the madness of it all. Those crazy SoCal kids.

One of the first occasions I realised that our food life was going to be different in Southern California was when we first arrived in LA and we were staying in a cheap motel on Sunset Boulevard. Just along from the Sunset Motel was the considerably more grand hotel, The Mondrian, where we could afford breakfast but not a room. We strolled early one morning and from somewhere out of the LA ether came the sound of Nils Lofgren singing 'Moon Tears' from the *Night*

After Night live album, a favourite of mine. Wow, this really is a rock'n'roll town I thought, as we were shown out on to a terrace which faced out across the low rise, palm tree strewn city. It sprawled west towards the sea, punctuated in the distance by some of the tall downtown office blocks. An early morning haze of heat and pollution made everything shimmer like maybe it wasn't actually real at all.

We had just sat down when into my peripheral vision strode a tall, rather thick set man who looked familiar. He was carrying an old vinyl Johnny Cash album under his arm. He turned and looked across to where we were seated. It was Peter Buck, guitarist for R.E.M., who at the time were riding high with their career defining album *Automatic for The People*. Cool.

Hey, it's LA. Of course you're having breakfast alongside one of the most prominent rock'n'roll musicians of the time. The second shock of the morning came when I opened the menu and saw it featured a tofu and vegetable 'scramble.' This might not seem much in 2011, but back then it was amazing that anywhere outside of a worthy vegetarian cafe would even think of serving such a thing. It was as though it was a normal part of life. Wow. At last we were being catered for and it felt good.

For that whole year we enjoyed the coolest of lifestyles and food was very much part of it. That remained the case every time we subsequently spent time on the west coast. One time we'd taken a trip up the Pacific Coast Highway and stopped off in Ventura, a posh little town just north of LA, finding a vegan restaurant we'd heard about.

We walked into this fantastic little wooden, flat board, green haven. It was staffed, as such places in California almost always are, by good-looking twenty-somethings in loose fitting non-sexist clothing. It seemed so relaxed and hip, with a mixture of upscale ethnic decoration and green foliage. Just lovely and very different from the frugal, stripped bare, wholefood, vegan establishment you might find in the UK which all too often for our liking took a hair-shirt approach to everything.

We went north to San Francisco where we went to a brilliant vegetarian, organic restaurant called The Millennium on Geary Street. It was upscale and as posh as you like. Tablecloths and everything.

We enjoyed an exquisite five-course meal which was everything such food wasn't in the UK. Light, subtly spiced and very original. It was such a hip place to eat in. It made being a non-meat eater so cool.

In San Luis Obispo we went to a place called Santa Veggie, which was a Chinese restaurant that had a vegan menu. This was like nothing we'd ever tasted. Essentially they used meat substitutes to recreate all manner of dishes that would normally be meat. It was incredible eating an eel made out of ... well, who knows, a mixture of various seaweeds and soya I think. This was part of a Buddhist Chinese tradition and was quite mind-blowing, so different, so not the sort of thing we'd been brought up with. It felt like progress in every sense of the word.

Hell, you could even get soya lattes in Starbucks before Starbucks was even heard of over here.

It is such positive experiences that bind you to your cultural choices. There was no doubt at all that we considered we had made not just the healthy or morally correct choice but also the cool choice too. California confirmed that and I'm sure that many who come to the lifestyle today also feel like the same.

We had our first taste of soya bacon on the west coast. You could grill this stuff until it was crispy and it was delicious. It was the start of a decade of fast food soya products.

Previously, you were pretty much restricted to dry burger mixes to which you added water. They were OK but tasted a bit like mashed up cardboard. Eventually a range of burgers and sausages started to become available that were much more like the real thing.

So we ate lots of soya burgers and sausages and roasts. We totally loved them. They were often flavoured with MSG and were just about the most contrived, processed foodstuff you could wish to encounter. They sounded very healthy and we thought they were – remember, they have no cholesterol and less fat than meat.

We continued to guzzle litres and litres of soya milk every week as well as lots of pulses, wholewheat, brown rice, soya oil and vegetables. Oh we were so bloody healthy it'd make you sick, ironically enough considering what happened later.

As the 1990s went on and we returned to the UK, food got, in real terms, cheaper and cheaper, so despite the fact that we were almost always skint, we could still afford to buy more and more food. Every supermarket was now stocking some sort of veggie/vegan sausages, burger, mince and even 'fish' cakes. We hadn't considered giving up the veggie lifestyle. Not once. As the years went on it became 'healthier' and more accepted as being very good for you. So much so that I doubt any medical professional would now suggest otherwise. They'd come around to our way of thinking. We had won.

But the very moment we should have been celebrating the mainstream's acceptance of some of the ideas we had held as truth for nearly thirty years, was the very moment we realised that our way of thinking had been utterly misguided, deluded and stubbornly destructive.

That choice to stop eating meat made so long ago, born out of a rebellion against my upbringing, psychedelic drugs and a counter-culture sensibility, had messed us up badly.

I was fat, exhausted, had very high cholesterol and was suffering from crippling IBS. I was falling apart and heading into middle age feeling well past my best and it was, frankly, bloody depressing.

Your lesson here is that oldest of adages, get it printed on a T-shirt, hell, I'll even print it on a T-shirt for you: Never Trust a Hippy.

We had been wrong and it was time to do something about it.

KILLING YOURSELF TO LIVE

We were walking past the Art Institute of Chicago on South Michigan Avenue, when I had an almighty gut spasm. It flooded my body with pain; a cold pain that made me sweat like a Geordie with a non-alcoholic beer.

It was a typical IBS incident. I knew I had very little time to get to a toilet, perhaps as little as two minutes, so I sprinted up the steps and into the huge, imposing building. Trouble was you had to pay to get in and use the toilets and there was a big queue with security checks to get through. The clock was ticking; I didn't have time to wait. I could see the toilets straight ahead, so I ran up to a large female security guard who stood alongside the booth to stop anyone getting in free.

Like almost all security staff and law enforcers in America, she was crammed into an uncomfortable, two sizes too small polyester uniform, the seams of which were stretched to capacity by seemingly limitless thick folds of fat, making it look as though it had shrunk on her while she was wearing it. Surely she'd have to be cut out of it at the end of the working day?

She placed a hand on her gun as I ran up, presumably looking red-faced, sweaty and distressed. Was I some sort of terrorist? She looked at me with the kind of haughty disdain that I'd only seen before on the faces of guests on *Ricki Lake*. In trying circumstances in America I always find it best to assume a Hugh Grant-like accent. It's no good talking in my Teesside accent because they just think I'm Australian or Dutch and that was no use. I needed to be readily identified as English and therefore a bit of a good egg. In my experience most Americans think the English have got lovely manners and are ever so polite, even though all our men are prone to homosexuality.

'Err … excuse me madam,' I said, doing my Hugh Grant thing, 'I find myself in a rather embarrassing situation. It really is most urgent that I use the restrooms. I am in, what I simply must call, some degree of digestive distress.'

Try this approach, if nothing else it's very good fun. You can act like every English gentleman you've ever seen in movies. If not Hugh Grant then Roger Moore or even Terry-Thomas if you have a bit of the rascal in you. We all know how to do it and they don't know that we're putting it on because they think *Mary Poppins* is a contemporary documentary about English society.

'You have to queue,' she said, pointing to the booth with a short but very fat finger. How do you put weight on your fingers? Has the fat filled up everywhere else and so has to bulge out the fingers as a last resort? Given how much we use our fingers, don't they burn off the fat? Not in Chicago it seemed.

I didn't have time to ponder such matters.

'Yes, yes, quite and rightly so, but this is very, very urgent. If I wait, I will quite assuredly be making an absolutely awful mess of this expensive marble floor and I'd hate to do that. Could I just run through without queuing?'

I pointed to the restrooms which were separated from me by one of those lines of detachable tape and pole affairs.

'I wouldn't ask but it really is a pressing matter.'

She looked at me with an expressionless face, as though trying to work out if this was some elaborate hoax. Clearly, I didn't look like a terrorist and even if I was, I had such nice manners. So she unhooked the roped off area and ushered me through.

'Bless you,' I said and ran to the toilets at top speed. As I flew, I could hear her laughter echoing behind me but there was no time left. I was seconds from deploying that most unwanted of verbs – brown-trousering.

I zoomed into the gents – thankfully American public toilets in such buildings are nothing like their British versions. They are big and clean. So big and clean you could move into them, hang a picture on the wall and set up home. Were they available to rent in West London they would cost £4,000 per week.

Consequently, you don't have to inspect ten cubicles to find one that is acceptable. In a single move I had removed trousers and underpants and was already in full explosive form as I descended onto the pan.

I had made it with a second to spare. I was sodden with sweat. I had to laugh out loud as I sat there. It had been like some sort of game show challenge.

As I left, I stopped to thank the security guard again. 'You're welcome, I hope you get better soon,' she said, kindly, now looking much more sympathetic as I'd proved to be an incontinent, possibly gay English dude – an arse-onist possibly, but not a terrorist.

This sort of incident was entirely typical and had become part of my regular life.

I should advise you in advance that this chapter is a bit messy and unpleasant. IBS isn't a nice condition to suffer from and it largely involves what we might call arse-based issues. I won't dwell on them overly but I do need to go into some detail. So get a stiff drink if you are of a squeamish disposition. Nurse! The screens, please.

To those who've never suffered from it, IBS probably sounds a fairly innocuous, trivial thing. A bit of digestive discomfort, well who doesn't get that from time to time? It might even sound like one of those made-up conditions that hypochondriacs might talk themselves into believing they have. After all, everyone is 'intolerant' of something these days. It's almost fashionable. I know, I know. I've heard it all over the years. However, if you've ever had it, you'll know just how miserable it can make you feel, not just occasionally but pretty much all of the time. In fact, it's so bad that starving yourself, simply not eating, is almost preferable than having to suffer another bout of it post-meal.

Yet for the first few years of being veggie I felt no side effects at all other than occasionally appalling wind, which I presumed was due to the high intake of lentils and beans, which is every vegetarian's heritage.

But around 1994 this all began to change. We'd returned to live in Harrogate after living in Laguna Beach. While on the west coast I was running on the beach every day but consuming more food than at any other time in life. The American-sized portion was a brilliant thing for kids from the north east of England, who had grown up poor and on meagre rations, and we indulged ourselves in the land of infinite food.

As I mentioned previously we'd also had access to all manner of new soya products which we couldn't get in the UK. Americans were well ahead of the UK in spotting the money to be made out of vegetarians and we loved them for it. We gorged ourselves all year long, eating soya in one form or another at virtually every meal. Then, as now, soya was sold as, and completely believed to be, very healthy.

It was protein without cholesterol and usually low in fat and calories.

Towards the end of our year there, I'd started to notice that after eating I would sometimes have a hard, distended stomach. I took no notice of it for ages. It didn't bother me much and I just thought it was the usual gas.

But gradually it got worse and was occasionally not just uncomfortable but actually painful. The top of my belly would buzz and it felt heavy, as though I'd eaten a really big meal even when I hadn't. Soon I began to have comedic, but quite hideous, explosive bowel movements.

This started to become a more regular event when we returned to the UK and within a year it was affecting me most days of most weeks. My diet was still low fat, high fibre, packed with vegetables and soya.

This as yet undiagnosed condition was really getting me down. So I went to the doctors and confessed the grisly symptoms. He hadn't a bloody clue. He thought it might be a consequence of drinking real ale. Not a good guess. He literally had nothing else to offer except an idea that 'it'll probably go away on its own'. Quite what he based this diagnosis on I have no idea. Actually, I do. He just fucking made it up! And he made it up because he didn't really consider it a serious condition.

So I walked away none the wiser. I stopped drinking real ale but it made no difference. Rather, it got worse. Between 1996 and 1998 the symptoms intensified; on occasions it was so hard for me to control my bowels at all that I was forced to dash into pubs and cafés to use toilets. The post-meal bloating began to happen after every single meal no matter what I ate and I began to get terrible indigestion, especially after eating bread, sometimes lying in bed with acid reflux burning my throat. I was always tired in the afternoons, suffered from headaches every day (as I always had done on this diet) and even a short walk would both tire me out and make my legs ache. Physically I was weak and I was becoming a mess.

After every meal I felt so heavy. Not just full but as though a large lead weight was in my belly, which would be distended and sore. This would last for two hours or more. Even a light meal brought this on. I couldn't understand what the matter was. It drove me crazy. It was all consuming. It was torture knowing you had to eat but also knowing what eating would do to you.

The diarrhoea was getting worse and worse. It'd start as soon as I got up and continue – in the worst periods – all day with up to seven or eight bowel movements passing a burning slurry of semi-digested food and mucus. At times it was so severe that I was having the anal equivalent of the dry heaves as there was nothing left to come out of me. I'd sit doubled up on the toilet in a cold sweat, racked in pain. I couldn't sit down after these episodes. Talk about a burning ring of fire. Frankly, it made me so bad tempered I'd have shot a man in Reno just to watch him die.

In 1999 I went to a new doctor who ran tests to see if I had Crohn's disease or if I was a coeliac and intolerant to gluten. But it came back negative. So then it was time for the endoscopy, which is essentially a camera on a stick put up your backside. He was worried I might have something growing up there. I was worried about him sticking that thing up there to find out.

It's always struck me as decidedly odd that anyone would want to be a proctologist. I mean, who among us feels the burning desire to peer up strangers' fundaments? I suppose I'm glad someone does but it is an undignified business and the suspicion remains that you are in the hands of a pervert.

Perhaps if he had a sense of humour it would have helped but he didn't; he was sour-faced, as perhaps was his prerogative given what he's doing for a living. Don't it make your brown eyes blue?

If you have never undergone this procedure, you are bound, like me, to be somewhat tense about it, which of course doesn't help as you go into camel-in-a-sandstorm mode. However, don't worry, it's really not as bad as you might imagine in advance. If, unlike me, you have a friendly and communicative doctor doing it, I'm sure it'd be even easier to deal with. It doesn't hurt.

There I am on the bed in the surgery, lying on one side and suddenly I feel the cold metal enter me like an alien probe. Could they not warm it? The thing they don't tell you is that after the initial shock, it's actually quite pleasurable. Yeah, who's the pervert now? I had the feeling that I shouldn't have told the doctor this. It's probably unethical or even illegal for a doctor to administer pleasure with an endoscope, but I figured hey, if a strange man has got to stick something up you then why not get what you can out of it? Whatever gets you through the night, or indeed the morning, in the surgery is my motto.

He probed me with the studious silence of a stamp-collector looking through albums for Penny Blacks. He had a good look around, or as good a look around as you can have of a bum hole and associated tubing, but found nothing of concern. As he pulled the endoscope out suddenly it felt as if my entire innards were going to come out with it. Blimey. It was most unpleasant and confirmed my long-held view that backdoor lovin' was not my idea of a good time.

It was good to know there was nothing cancerous in there but once again the medical man couldn't offer a diagnosis as to what was causing this condition nor how to stop it and so he essentially gave up. He wouldn't admit to giving up but the fact was he had no further solutions to offer, so he sent me to a 'specialist' at a small local hospital.

This was a bit of a joke really. When you're told someone is a specialist, you expect them to have more knowledge than your average doctor don't you? Certainly more than a drunken man in the street. I'm not sure the man I saw could make such a claim. Perhaps he was just a drunken man in the street masquerading as a specialist. I actually hope so.

For a start, he looked older than God. And given IBS is such a modern condition I immediately wondered if he was bang up to date with his reading on the subject. It seemed more than likely that he wasn't. By his age you're usually more concerned with your own bowels, not those of some stranger.

Still you've waited bloody months for this consultation so you go with it just on the off chance that he's a genius and is hiding his innate brilliance behind a veneer of bumbling ineptitude.

But of course, he isn't a genius, he's actually just an old bloke who doesn't have a clue what is wrong.

He peered at my bum hole and actually drew it on a bit of paper. Maybe he collected bum-hole drawings for his 'arses I have known' collection. After this sketch he put his finger up me. Just the one. I was getting used to this type of violation by now and was much less tense.

'Hmm you're a bit inflamed,' he said, which, frankly, anyone could have diagnosed without inserting a finger up my bottom. Of course I'm inflamed. Tell me something I don't know, pal. I'm shitting for Britain and what's more, I'm winning.

At first he wanted to put me in hospital just 'to keep

an eye on me'. 'These things often clear up after a spell in hospital,' he said. Why? Is hospital food some sort of cure-all panacea? I was furious. Bugger off, I thought. You're talking rubbish. He couldn't give me any reasons as to why this might happen. He was just guessing like anyone who isn't a 'specialist' would guess. What the hell was the use of sitting in a hospital bed?

I thought this would be a waste of public money. There was no offer of specific treatment if I did sit in a hospital, all the while risking catching even more unpleasant diseases. I also worked for myself so didn't have time to take off work on the sick.

So instead of a spell on the local ward he gave me something called Fibrogel which he said would 'bind your stools together'.

I immediately thought this was an idiotic notion because had he looked at my diet diaries he'd have realised I ate more fibre than a horse. Remember I'm eating brown rice, wholemeal bread and a dozen portions of fruit and veg a day. No human on earth was eating more fibre than me. If my stools were going to be solidified by fibre they already would have been. But he didn't listen to me and preferred only to hear his own misinformed ignorance. I'm only the patient, what could I know about it, eh?

So much of my contact with doctors was like this. Talking to themselves, not listening to me and then going down some prescribed route regardless of how appropriate it was to me.

Stupidly, stupidly, stupidly, I didn't trust my own instincts and went along with this madness hoping that perhaps he knew what he was talking about. But he was an idiot and his prescription little short of torture. The Fibrogel induced some of the most violent reactions I have ever suffered from.

I took it twice and it sent me onto a new level of gross-out symptoms as I passed the entire contents of my body into the toilet in a constant stream of jellified slurry, my guts in spasm and my whole body in a cold sweat. The pain was awful and the burning so intense it was impossible to sit down as it felt as though I was sitting on hot coals. It brought me to tears. These incidents left me exhausted and wrung out.

One episode saw me passing out what I can only describe as a thick foam of shit and mucus, which looked like a Mars bar had been put in a food processor with some washing up liquid and agitated vigorously. I looked at the miasma that had recently been inside of me with a mixture of disgust and awe at the volume of heinous effluent that you can expunge. It was like looking at a Jackson Pollock painting made from my own bodily fluids. Radical art perhaps, but a bloody awful way of life.

It was as though my whole body was in revolt. It was certainly revolting. Utterly offensive. We tend to have a high tolerance for our own foulness don't we? Who doesn't like the smell of their own farts? But this was something else. It was loathsome and rank; like rotting from the inside out. It made me hate my body for going wrong. I was utterly disgusted.

I cursed the old fool and vowed not to have anything to do with doctors again. They were making things much, much worse and wasting my valuable time.

I began to do more research and I could see that quite clearly my symptoms fell under the broad banner of Irritable Bowel Syndrome. Equally obviously, it seemed likely that it was provoked by something I was eating. But what was it?

I began to omit specific foods from my diet but to no effect at all. I removed lentils and beans. Then I stopped drinking beer, then all alcohol. It had no effect. I had a period not eating wheat. Then I tried not eating gluten. I stopped eating brown rice. I tried not eating brassica such as cabbage and broccoli. I cut out fruit. None of these exclusions made any difference.

For various periods of time across ten years I stopped eating yeast, I laid off eggs and dairy, I drank lots of water, I stopped drinking alcohol, I tried white bread and white rice and a low fibre diet. Nothing worked. I still had the same conditions. The condition remained and was with me all the time, day after day, month after month year after year.

And the ill health didn't stop with IBS. In the process of doing blood tests it was discovered I had very high cholesterol. A reading of 9.2 the doctor said with a face like thunder. It felt as though I was morally lacking to have this reading. As though I'd acquired it through mugging pensioners or something. He showed me a graph which he said illustrated the increased likelihood that I'd have a heart attack due to this high level of cholesterol and suggested I go on the then new wonder drug statins to reduce this possibility.

He didn't question why or how this level was so high. He knew it couldn't have been dietary related because I hadn't eaten any cholesterol for years and years. He told me that only 30 per cent of your cholesterol is from your diet anyway – where my 30 per cent had gone he didn't explain. Given my dad had gone tits up with the heart attack I naturally agreed to take 40mg of Lipitor for the rest of my bloody life. This was just further confirmation that I was a mess. That I was falling apart. It was very depressing.

In 2005 we moved to Edinburgh, Scotland's capital and a place of immense history and culture. I thought I'd approach a local GP with my problems. After all, surely the finest medical minds would be here in this city of learning. And IBS was now a well-known and recognised condition that many people were suffering from. Surely, a progressive GP would know more than me about this and be able to help.

Could she bollocks.

In common with all the others, she couldn't offer any help at all. It was suggested I try various IBS tablets from Boots as though I wouldn't have tried them already. I had tried everything. Why wouldn't I have? But they hadn't worked. She suggested lots of other things that I had already tried ten years ago. She started to suggest keeping a food diary but I interrupted her, 'Look, I've been through all this now for years. I've kept food diaries, I've tried exclusion diets and nothing has made it better.'

She looked at me haughtily, as though I was overreacting, at which point, given the digestive distress brewing inside of me, I could have literally pooed on her desk. Maybe I should have done so to make my point.

I just wish a GP could say these words, 'I really don't know what's causing this. I don't have a clue. Do you have any ideas?'

Don't try and pretend you have any bloody idea when you don't. I don't care that you don't know; I understand that you can't know everything and that learning has a finite limit, but don't pretend to have knowledge that you clearly don't have and then don't sneer at me when I mention I've researched my condition as though I am some sort of hypochondriac. All of which I felt from this particular doctor. As soon as you hear them say 'Did you read that on the internet?' you know the discussion is over.

The last time I went to the doctor's surgery about my IBS was to see a young woman called 'The Nutritionist'. I thought it'd be interesting to see exactly what she would say. So I kept her a food diary for a couple of weeks and presented it to her, full, as per usual, of brown rice, nuts, lentils, olive oil, garlic, a dozen portions of fruit and veg a day, tofu and soya milk. Not an ounce of cholesterol, low in fat, very low in saturated fat, low in sugar, high in fibre. Laughably so.

She sat there in silence and looked at the diary. Obviously, she could find nothing whatsoever in it to criticise. Mind you, in truth she didn't exactly exude scholarly learning, coming across as little more than a student who has just scraped through some easy degree. I recognised this look because I have it myself having got a BA (Hons.) second-class degree despite not reading more than one course book from cover to cover in three years.

She had absorbed a set of basic notions and rather than look for alternatives or think outside of the box her education had put her in – even though that education offered no insight into what was wrong with me – she just repeated those notions regardless of the facts that were before her. From what she was reading I shouldn't have been fat, let alone clinically obese. She just looked back at me, embarrassed that I was a wobbly contradiction of her learning. I think she just assumed I was lying.

To help excuse her I suggested that I must simply be eating too large a portion of these healthy foods, after all, a big bowl of brown rice contains a lot of calories. This was probably true. It's really easy to over eat carbs. She wasn't keen to agree with this, probably because she had been taught calories from brown rice are good calories and calories from fat are bad. It was quite funny really. Failing to find anything in the diary, she started telling me all the foods I shouldn't eat, even though, clearly, I didn't actually eat any of them.

She assumed I ate sugar, which I almost never did. She assumed I ate cakes and biscuits, which I almost never did. She assumed I ate chocolate, which I almost never did. She assumed I regularly ate chips, which I almost never did. She assumed all of these things, warned me not to eat them and then looked on in amazement when I said, 'Look, I really don't eat like that. I'm an old school healthy food hippy. I was eating healthy food since before you were born, darlin'.'

'There are a lot of calories in nuts,' she proffered meekly.

'Yes, but they're my main source of first-class protein,' I countered – wrongly as it happened as nuts are not a first-class protein or at least, not a complete protein. You'd have thought she'd have corrected me.

She started trying to tell me not to eat butter as it was full of cholesterol which, even as she said it, was an outdated view of the role of cholesterol but I stopped her mid-sentence and told her flatly, 'I have never in my whole adult life eaten butter. I have barely eaten any cholesterol since 1984!'

She looked blankly at me, not computing this fully.

It must not have occurred to her to question my vegetarianism, possibly out of some PC guidelines not to insult the patient's beliefs or more likely because she'd been taught it was a healthier regime than 'normal' diets.

She clearly had reached the end of her knowledge so I made my excuses and left her. She was 100 per cent useless, as I knew she would be, but it wasn't her fault really. She was just sticking to the party line just like all the doctors. It's a shame there isn't room for more independent and adventurous thinking in the health service, be it with doctors or nutritionists or whomever, especially when the conventional advice has failed to improve the patient. What's to lose?

For years and years both Dawn and I tried to get the NHS to help us get well. We gave them every chance to find out what was wrong with us. But they didn't and they couldn't. They never got near, never had a clue and didn't even seem to have any imagination about how to treat either of us.

It was so frustrating because eventually you begin to feel it's actually your own fault that they don't know what's going on. Time and again I got a flippant, offhand attitude from doctors as I dismissed their suggestions about diet or lifestyle simply because I had tried them all many times previously to no effect. It definitely annoyed them. I know this might have been because I can be, appropriately enough, an arsey sod. And I'm not always great at the social niceties. But hellfire, I never insulted any of them, and some gave me good reason to. And after all, I was in constant pain and discomfort for nearly twenty years – I had reason to be grumpy: I was sitting on a volcano. I only went to the doctors because I was desperate. It really was a last resort. I just hoped they'd have some ideas I'd overlooked. But they didn't even have the ones I'd tried and failed with. It was as though I was on chapter 49 of a 50 chapter book and they were still reading the introduction.

Eventually, it seemed to me that they laid the blame for the situation onto the patient, as though their ignorance is your fault. 'What would you like me to do for you?' they would say, with a tinge of 'You're just being awkward, please sod off' about it after I'd replied 'Tried that, it didn't work,' to all their suggestions. Well, what do you think Sherlock? I'd like you to use some medical knowledge to find out what's wrong with me? That is your gig, right?

Sorry I don't have a more easily treatable disease. Of course it was my fault for eating a diet that destroyed me from the inside out but I have to say that their performance en masse by any standards was an abject, pitiful failure. Because the fact is, there was research out there which could have guided them to a solution. It might not have been in their medical text books but since those text books had failed to deliver a solution why not consider them? There were plenty of tests that could have been done that were not. I just didn't know about them at the time – but they should have.

My impression was that it was never really taken seriously as a condition and I often felt they thought I was some sort of hypochondriac. This is not how it should be. Once the standard treatments are exhausted, there should be more imagination, more experimental, more out-of-the-box thinking. But this seemed beyond everyone's remit. Indeed, throughout this fiasco, I felt the main concern for everyone was to cover their backs and not do anything that might rock the boat. Even though I was sick, that seemed much less important than following The Path.

Having seen many practitioners over many years in several different parts of the country, it has been like dealing with the same doctor each time, as though one is a replica of the other. All spew out the same learning in the same way regardless of what you say. There appears to be no individual thinking, no intelligence applied specifically to you. Just lists of boxes to tick and The Stuff We Do In Situations Like This. And there is nothing else if that fails. Slowly, slowly, slowly, they crush your spirit and leave you still sick. Worse still, it all takes so bloody long. A week for a blood test, two more weeks to see the doctor for five minutes, then another week for another blood test and another week or two for your next five minutes with the GP, all of which reveals nothing so then you get sent to a specialist which takes two months to happen. They take two minutes and decide you need another blood test. Then you wait two or three weeks for the results of that test to be sent to your doctor. It reveals nothing. It's taken over three months for less than fifteen minutes of treatment or consultation and you are no further forward. So the whole process starts over again, ad infinitum, with more tests and different specialists who all too often do not seem that special.

This is your life once you get on the NHS treadmill. It would be tempting to suggest that it is a system set up to keep everyone involved in work rather than efficiently deliver health solutions.

Can't it at least be quicker? Why, when a doctor says, right, we'll do a blood test, can't they just take the blood there and then? Why do you have to wait a week for an appointment for someone else to take it? Surely any doctor can take blood? Is it any wonder when, after a year of this, you sit down still sick as a dog and feel a bit impatient and testy? No. Do you get sympathy? No. Instead they get sneery with you for trying to self-medicate or diagnose from your own research. Like that makes me a real bloody idiot doesn't it? Yeah, I'm such a dummy for trying to make myself better. Leave it to the highly paid professional instead, eh? Well it's just as well I didn't, isn't it, because they'd still be a highly paid professional and I'd still be fucking ill.

So I had given up on the NHS solutions and eventually I had all but given up trying to heal myself at home. I felt I'd tried everything: food exclusion, tablets, homeopathy, creams, potions, suppositories and herbal medicine. I had bought so many so-called cures and spent so much money for so long but to no lasting improvement.

I tried peppermint oil and peppermint tea, both of which are lovely but had no impact on my symptoms at all. I tried fennel tea too, again, a lovely brew but of no help. I tried almost every product that had probiotic written on it. Nada. The only thing that was effective in anyway was Diocalm, which would essentially slow my gut down so that I could go of out the house for an hour or three without having to plan a trip around toilet breaks. If I forgot to do this, I was in trouble.

It was essential when in public but it didn't cure me, of course, it just briefly alleviated the problem. Over-the-counter drugs such as Buscopan and Colofac as well as Boots' own brand of IBS drugs might as well have been Smarties for all the good they did. There really is no point in taking them because even if they take away some of your symptoms, until you address the underlying root cause of why you're suffering from IBS you are simply going to continue suffering from it. The drugs don't cure it and I suspect that's how the drug companies like it. If they cured it you'd have no reason to keep buying them.

No, the ideal pill from the pharmaceutical industry's point of view is one that gives some relief temporarily for a recurring condition. Thus you have to keep buying them in order to get that modest relief. But, as I say, I ate the things like sweets and felt not discernibly any different at all.

As if all of this wasn't bad enough, my body had one more cruel trick to play on me. By 2007 I had developed really bad haemorrhoids, undoubtedly brought on by fifteen years of ferocious digestive disorder. I could feel them moving during bowel movements. Over a period of around a year these got bigger and bigger and more painful. They'd throb and bring me out in a cold sweat. This is called stage two haemorrhoids.

I kept on passing shit like a waterfall and they got bigger and bigger and hurt like hell. Eventually they started to emerge after passing anything and I had to push them back in. This is called stage three. There are only four stages, the last being permanently hanging out your arse like a bunch of grapes in the classic, comedy style. I couldn't find any humour in the condition. It was so depressing. It was another physical manifestation of my dysfunctional body breaking down and going wrong. In some ways it was the worst thing of all because, all joking aside, it's happening to you in an intimate part of your body and it is absolutely fucking vile to have to deal with day after day, week after week.

At first, pushing them back in was easy, like pushing a

small grape up a pipe (if you have ever found yourself in a situation where you have to push a grape up a pipe, you'll already know what it's like). But as they swelled up bigger and bigger it got tougher to do and sometimes impossible – the more tense you get, your body goes into No Entry Allowed mode.

I knew where all this was headed. Stage four – being permanently external – and then they would need surgery because it would be impossible to live with. The pain would be just too much. This scared me. Who wants someone operating on your bum hole, after all?

But I didn't know what to do to stop it. I had failed to stop my IBS and it was surely that which was causing it. I felt utterly helpless. As with the IBS, all the proprietary creams and suppositories didn't help. In fact, at times I wonder if there is anything that chemists sell that actually does the job it purports to do. It often seems like modern medicine is one big con. If you look at the small print of many of these treatments, they insert the word 'can' in front of the medicinal claim. It is surely a get out clause. Pile cream is supposed to reduce 'swelling' and 'itching' but it didn't for me, not in the slightest, and if not for me, then for whom? Were my piles somehow atypical in being resistant to the brilliantly named Anusol? Did I somehow have an anti-Anusol arse?

My entrenched cynicism towards doctors meant I didn't bother seeking any GP help. It was pointless given I had researched my options and knew all the possibilities and all the treatments, and knew there was nothing they could tell me that I didn't already know. The official advice is to eat plenty of fibre, have lots to drink, take fibre supplements, avoid codeine and go to the toilet at the first urge. Yeah right, I did all that anyway. It was my life. Now tell me something that will help. Nada. As per usual.

I was just hoping that it would somehow get better. But I knew it wouldn't.

Then Dawn discovered a website that had an obscure old cure for haemorrhoids. Horse chestnuts! She found some tablets which contained extract from the seed of the horse chestnut tree. I joked that this was most appropriate as my piles were certainly the size of conkers. It sounds an unlikely cure doesn't it? There was little medical evidence to prove that this would work except for the assertion that it was a traditional old country cure. I didn't think for a moment that it would work but I had nothing to lose.

So I started taking them every day and of course they solved nothing. Three months of taking three tablets a day and I was still playing billiards with my piles every day. But Dawn's research said it could take up to six months to work and said I should keep taking them. So I did.

After four months, incredibly, she was proved right. One morning I woke up and passed a lot of blood. This is about as terrifying a thing that can come out of you and I've had a lot of pretty terrifying things come out of me. I peered down at the thick ribbons of bright red blood and an icy shard of mortality entered my heart. Something bad must have happened. This was the start of the end. I wasn't going to make fifty. I was dying.

However, as I began to clean myself up, I immediately noticed the piles had shrunk from the size of big grapes to the size of peas and were barely emerging. All that blood had to be from the piles. Was that good or bad? At first I didn't know but with a bit of research it seemed likely that this was what happened when they shrank and disappeared. The vein that has swollen up weakens and leaks and deflates Mr Grape. And so it proved. Over the next two days the blood steadily decreased and then stopped and the piles were gone.

As recommended, I kept taking them for six months and they totally disappeared outside and in. As it was the only change I'd made, I was certain it had to be the horse chestnut tablets that had worked. I couldn't see why it would have happened otherwise. Indeed, it seemed as if this was a condition usually only reversible under the knife.

It's worth bearing in mind that had I gone to the doctor, they would have sneered at horse chestnut tablets as not a clinically proved solution, as quackery. I would have been no better off and still suffering. So who was right and who was wrong? It's obvious to me.

This cure felt like a massive victory and offered the first proof that it was possible to improve your own health through self-diagnosis and treatment. It also proved to me that official advice on this was, at least for me, just redundant or inappropriate and that alternative solutions could work.

By 2008 I was fourteen and a half stone and as I'm only a medium build, it sat heavily. Sadly, getting rid of the piles didn't reduce my weight. But such is the way of these things I didn't really think I was actually quite as fat as I was. Somehow, because it happened slowly, I just took my expanded waistline as part of getting older. I didn't see myself as a fat bloke at all; my new fondness for elasticated waistbands was just because they were more practical.

In the New Year of 2008 we went for a month's break in California, a week of which was in Palm Springs. We'd rented a lovely, cool 1950s-style house with a pool and large gardens. The sort of gaff you'd have found Frank and Deano drinking martinis in the late 1950s. It was in the eighties every day and we'd eat al fresco beside the pool. During the course of doing so, we each took the usual holiday snaps.

When we were looking at the photos on our return I saw a picture of myself sitting at the table with my shirt off in the sun, a massive belly hanging off me like a ruck-sack, my top half wrapped in a blanket of fat. I looked like a well-lagged boiler.

I was really shocked. Perhaps you just don't really see yourself as you are when you look in the mirror because I hadn't really thought I was *that* fat, but the photo was living proof of it. The detached third-person viewpoint of the camera seemed to bring it home.

It's a weird feeling being offended by yourself, or at least it is for someone like me who isn't prone to too much self-loathing. But I looked at that and I thought, you fat bastard, you look just like your dad did. This was not a good thing, especially given how it ended for him on the sofa aged just sixty-five.

In fact, we'd both put so much weight on over the years that we were now struggling to walk up Edinburgh's many hilly streets without feeling breathless and tired out after-wards. It was pathetic really. Why were we doing this to ourselves? It wasn't as if getting fat was making life any more pleasurable or comfortable. We were complacent in our self-appointed healthy diet as though it offered protection from such a condition – clearly it hadn't.

So the week we came back, early in 2008, we resolved to do something about it. We bought a couple of bikes and started doing a ten-mile ride every weekend. At the same time we started to restrict calorie consumption radically. We did this primarily by reducing carbohydrates, especially potatoes, rice and bread and we cut fat intake back to a bare mini-mum. At the same time we reduced portion size. The weight dropped off right away. From February to December I went from fourteen and a half stone to under eleven; Dawn from nearly fourteen and a half to twelve. Even another month in Las Vegas in November didn't put a pound on us.

Losing weight is quite compulsive. You feel virtuous and the extra energy you have from not dragging a sack of fat around with you makes you feel good about yourself. But all the time, in the back of my mind I was worried that I would put weight back on when I returned to my 'normal' healthy diet. It would be impossible to exist on this starvation diet long term. I already felt light-headed and often suffered complete collapses of energy through lack of food, leaving me feeling weak and almost stoned – but not in a good way.

I was also suffering random, weird muscle pains, which felt like a really bad Chinese burn. This worried me a little as I suspected, rightly, that I was losing fat but also losing muscle and I didn't have that much to lose. I was in effect, wasting away. I actually had started to look quite gaunt, so much so that friends who hadn't seen me for a while thought I was anorexic. The fact was, although I was now thinner and had lost my big belly, I was weak and, although lighter, not robust. My body fat percentage was still quite high for my weight – around 25 per cent. I was what is sometimes called 'skinny fat'.

I realised that it was no good just being lighter; I really owed it to myself to be fitter and stronger because it would improve my quality of life.

Many men probably go through this around my age. However old you feel in your head, you have to accept you are not the man you once were; you are no longer the kid who could rock 'n' roll all night and party every day. I was going to seed and I knew it and I didn't like that feeling at all. Suddenly I felt the cold shudder of the grave – that sense of mortality that is everyone's destiny – and decided there and then that it was better to burn out than rust. It was time to get healthy, to get fit, to get stronger. I knew from that moment of realisation that this was the end of one way of life and the start of another – but I didn't yet know how.

During that jaunt to Las Vegas we were renting an apartment in The Signature at MGM Grand. Downstairs was a gym for residents. Neither of us had ever been in a gym. Especially not in Las Vegas. You do getting up late, you do 5am gambling sprees and you do drinking cocktails for breakfast. Your daily exercise is achieved by walking from the poker machines to the bar and back a few times every hour.

So we shuffled in rather self-consciously and sat on exercise bikes for an hour, pedalling away and sweating like a couple of hot pigs. It was OK though. The gym itself was very upmarket, with spotless equipment and even a maid service on hand to dispense towels and water!

So when we came home we thought we'd try to get fitter and try to get a bit stronger too so we joined a Bannatyne's just a minute from where we lived. We had wrongly assumed it would be full of finely honed athletic types, when in reality it was full of fat, sweaty Scottish people trying to shed the pounds built up eating pies. It was also, in comparison to the Vegas gym, manky and worn out. No towels, apples or spring water. In fact, I'm sure if it was proposed on *Dragons' Den* as a business Duncan would rip it to pieces mercilessly as not up to standard and say he was out.

Throughout this weight loss period my IBS improved slightly; I put this down to just eating a lot less, so I didn't feel as heavy or bloated all the time, though I was still keeping the sewage system busy.

While it was substantially better than the worst days of a few years previously, I was still a long way from being normal – in fact, I no longer had any memory of what 'normal' actually meant, so long had it been since I had enjoyed such a condition.

Dawn meanwhile was suffering with a whole host of problems. She had very congested sinuses, was always tired, had days when her mind was clouded and heavy, when she felt as though a shroud covered her. She'd get terrible headaches and generally felt listless and increasingly depressed and emotionally fragile.

She had gone to the doctor who merely kept prescribing nasal sprays and did so until her nose bled from over-using them. That was where the advice ended, until Dawn said she was depressed. Out came the Prozac prescription, which she ignored on the basis that she was depressed because she was ill and the way to relieve the depression was to relieve the illness. Isn't that just really bloody obvious? Not to the doctor in question, who as ever treated the symptoms and not the causes.

After months of waiting she was sent to an ear, nose and throat (ENT) 'specialist' who just took an X-ray of her sinuses – which revealed nothing. That was the extent of his specialness. Of course, it revealed nothing because her sinus congestion was manifestly an allergic reaction of some sort. Dawn suggested this and so was sent to another 'specialist' who tested for allergies to dust mites and cat fur etc. It seemed beyond anyone's comprehension that this could be an allergic reaction with its root in diet. It didn't occur to anyone. Indeed, one of the ENT specialists Dawn saw hadn't even heard of hormonal rhinitis, a condition which is documented on the NHS website and which could have been the cause. When you know more than the specialist, you inevitably lose faith in the system.

So it was back to the doctor for a lot of vacant looks and not much else. All of this specialist treatment had taken a remarkable six months for two three-minute appointments. Proof, if it were needed, that if you are not proactive in helping yourself, you'll be dead before they get round to working anything out, which is maybe what they want. It makes the waiting lists shorter.

It all take a ridiculous length of time and it's so depressing having to go to a hospital for such tests, if only because you've got to get through the small, ragged army of papery-skinned, death-warmed-up people in their pyjamas and nighties standing outside smoking as though it was the stuff of life rather than death. For independently minded, self-motivated people, in my experience the NHS is utterly draining. It requires you to sit there in silence like a dumb-ass fuckwit, for an undetermined length of time (your time is of no importance to anyone once you enter the NHS), just a number in the system, another blank-eyed drone in the hospital hive.

Who you are is now irrelevant. Just shut up and wait for the person in the white coat to hand a diagnosis down from on high like the soulless, slack-jawed sap you are. I loathe it.

I don't have any solutions as to how to make things better but there's got to be a superior way; everyone involved from nurses upwards treats every person as though they are barely sentient and possibly senile, which to be fair, describes some of the people there very well. So maybe that is appropriate most of the time, but please don't treat me like that.

Then one day Dawn dropped a massive bombshell; not one of those small bombshells, oh no, this was a proper, big nuclear bombshell.

'We should eat meat,' she said, flatly.

The words made me go as cold as ice. Her words were a freezing bolt of electricity. My first response was the obvious one.

'Why?'

'Because all our health issues are being caused not just by what we are eating but also by what we're not eating. Not eating meat is the problem,' she said, enigmatically, as is her wont.

Fucking hell, I thought. But, but, but... I'm not a meat eater.

I fought against the idea for days, wrestling with it in my mind. The idea hurt my sense of personal identity and challenged my whole moral and political outlook. Perhaps even more than that, it meant changing habits built up over twenty-six years. I had a comfortable, default position and it meant ditching that and starting out on a new path. That intimidated me and made me resist it initially but was actually also what finally persuaded me to do it. It was something new and different and even though I didn't really want to admit it to myself for a while, that was quite exciting. A new, meaty vista to explore was intriguing.

I mulled it over for a few days. I knew that it made sense. Or at the very least, it was an option I hadn't tried in order to get well. I'd done everything else to no effect. The IBS continued to ravage my digestive system regardless.

I kept asking myself, 'Have you given up? Are you just going to live the rest of your life like this?'

One part of me said yes. I had given up. It had been seventeen bloody years of illness. It was all I knew. It was my daily life. I was used to it. I had little memory of what it was like to eat and not feel heavy and bloated. I planned my life around easy and quick access to toilets. I coped. People cope with far worse conditions, I knew that. I didn't even imagine that there was a life not just without IBS but a happier, more content life out there with more energy, greater mental acuity and strength. That didn't even occur to me.

The thought of eating bloody, dead animals was so physically scary as well as psychologically and philosophically intimidating but, then again, what if it worked? Would it really be so bad? People I liked and respected ate meat. They were not demons. They also did not have a clown's misfiring car for an arse.

After a few days, Dawn declared that she was going to do it, regardless of whether I did or not. She didn't put any pressure on me to follow suit. But we've always done everything together and this was such a big thing that the fact she was going to do it anyway pushed me over the edge. I could just try it once or twice. Just to see if it made any difference. I could always go back to being a vegan after this experiment.

The truth is I gave up my vegetarian principles quite quickly and easily once I'd got over the initial shock of the very idea. I've since wondered if this actually meant that it was more of a habit than a principle and that I'm actually quite emotionally and morally shallow. Maybe it's not for me to judge. But it seems likely. I should have been dragged kicking and screaming into the butchers but I just wasn't. I thought, sod it, let's just do it and see what happens. What's the worst that could happen?

To be really honest, I didn't believe it would make any difference to my health. Not really. Because nothing had.

We. Would. Eat. Meat.

So we looked up the nearest organic farm shop to us, found one just outside of Edinburgh in the Scottish borders and set out to buy our first products of slaughter since 1984. As we took off I was excited and really looking forward to it. It was all new, a journey into the unknown and who knew where it might lead?

I couldn't have imagined how completely it would change me – physically, mentally and emotionally. I was looking forward to embracing a new culture and thought about how many great restaurants would no longer be out of bounds to us. I would never have thought that this trip, this mere twenty-five-mile journey would be such a profound one and would change my life completely. It's strange really. You never know what the future holds. You assume how life has been in the past will be how it is going to be in the future. I thought eating meat would be just like my life not eating meat but with, well, added meat. I was wrong. I was about to be transformed from a sick, shitty, weak bloke into someone with a lust for life.

I was about to undergo the Meat Fix.

TWO AGAINST NATURE

Our big decision to buy – and eat – meat confirmed, we set off to Whitmuir Farm, an organic farm shop on the Scottish borders, and into uncharted territory. I had literally no idea how you bought meat. Of course I knew you paid money for it; I wasn't expecting to have to barter in some medieval way, no. What I mean is to my eyes it all looked like red or pink flesh with fat attached.

I couldn't tell the difference between one bloody lump and another. I had no reason to know. How did you know which cut was which and what gigot, sirloin and brisket meant? I couldn't tell the difference between pork and lamb. I didn't know a fillet steak from rib-eye. I wasn't even sure I knew which was lamb and which was beef. It was all red and it was all bleeding. I also had no idea how much meat one ate in a sitting. A hundred grams? Two hundred? Five hundred? What amount of meat should you eat? It was all a mystery – after all, it was so long since I'd bought any, so long, in fact, that we now had to buy it in pounds and ounces, not grams.

As we walked into the farm shop I half expected an alarm to go off and the woman behind the counter to point to us, shake her head and say, 'I'm sorry sir, I can't serve you. You're a vegetarian and you don't believe in animals being killed for food. These are all corpses you know, they're not soya meat.'

It really did feel that illegal. It seemed like we must surely stand out in some way, as though we had big green Vs on our foreheads.

But no alarms went off and they merely assumed we were regular people here to buy organic meat. If only they knew. I felt acutely self-conscious: an enormous meat-based social faux pas was surely about to happen.

A long, refrigerated unit housed all the cuts and joints. I wandered over and took a look at the display of various beef, lamb, mutton and chicken. It was, inescapably, chopped up animals of some description. Could have been humans for all I knew. There was no hiding the bloody fact but weirdly, perhaps, that is what I wanted to see. I had no interest in buying something sanitised and pre-prepared to pretend it was anything else except a slaughtered beast. If I was going to eat meat then I wanted to test my feelings about it. I wanted to be exposed to the full, gory story. I didn't want to be a pussy about it. I wanted to face it. If you're going to effectively sanction a creature's death you really should metaphorically shake hands, or hooves or paws with it.

So, what to buy? I tried to recollect what I used to like to eat as a kid. I knew I had loved liver but had no idea if it was lamb's, calf's or ox liver, all of which were on display here. I opted entirely at random for some ox liver. It looked like purple jelly. We also bought rib-eye steaks, minced beef and a large bag of bones to make stock with. The bones were free – clearly fantastic value – but they were big beef bones, dripping blood and wrapped in fat and bits of flesh. Yup, this was definitely an animal; either that or some very sophisticated textured vegetable protein.

My palms were a bit sweaty, fearful of the dead flesh, as though it might sit up and say 'Hey, son, what the hell are you doing eating me? It bloody well hurts you know.'

But, as I say, this was quite deliberately a test of attitude and feelings. Was this change in eating just a silly fad that we were both entertaining or had we really had a more profound change of heart? Even as I bought the meat I thought Dawn certainly had, but I still didn't really know. To be honest, at that moment I couldn't see this being something I really wanted to take part in long term. I was putting a brave face on it, but carrying dismembered animals in a bag wasn't filling me with much joy.

As we drove the twenty-five miles back home it felt as though we had committed a crime, not that I know what that feels like, honestly.

Obviously, having bags of meat in the car is an entirely normal thing for most of the population; entirely unexceptional in fact although perhaps a carrier bag of bones was less common. But we realised as we travelled that we'd only got a car in 1987, three years into being veggie, so we'd never had meat in the car before. It all added to the sense of weird unfamiliarity about the situation.

As we took the bags of meat in to the house, I knew the most challenging part lay ahead: cooking the bleeding flesh.

As we unwrapped it all we were both intimidated but Dawn said, 'Look, people have been eating meat since the dawn of time, what makes us think we should be so different? These animals have been organically, locally reared, fed naturally, they were slaughtered locally and have probably had as good a life as any cow could have in the time it was alive.'

Her words had some sense but I still couldn't really shake the feeling that it seemed unfair on the beast to kill it to eat it.

But sod it, I had decided to try eating meat and once I've made my mind up to do something I'm damn well going to do it.

I googled how to cook liver, because after twenty-six

years I really couldn't remember, printed out a recipe and went to the kitchen.

Opening the packet of liver was like being at the scene of some terrible accident. Blood was everywhere!

'Just follow the fucking recipe you wuss,' I kept telling myself as I mopped the oozing organ with kitchen paper to dry off the excess blood. It looked like a murder scene. In a way, I suppose it was. I found myself holding my breath and then only breathing through my mouth so I wasn't able to smell it, not that it smelled especially strongly. I cut it into slices, feeling all the while like some sort of brutal surgeon. I heated some oil and put the slices into the pan. As they sizzled, more blood oozed out of them, as though the thing was still alive, its heart still pumping blood through its veins. It was as though it still had life, some kind of accusatory giblet.

'Just cook it, just bloody cook it, eat it and get this over with,' I kept telling myself.

The recipe said to cook it until it was still pink but I couldn't face that at all, I didn't want a trace of uncooked blood in my mouth so I fried it until it was very brown. I knew this meant it would be hard and rubbery but sod it, that was how it always was when I was a child.

It smelled very familiar, it smelled of animal and it took me right back to the last time I'd cooked and eaten liver when we were living on the Black Isle in 1984, when I used to regularly cook us a cracking liver and onions in thick gravy. It was so good that Dawn, previously not a liver lover, was converted to its pleasures.

I fried some onions as a nod to that old tradition and to give me something familiar to eat with the liver. I sat down to bite into it. I looked at it. Once cooked it looked fairly innocuous. It could have been soya meat, in fact.

I'd like to say that there was a chorus of angels, or butchers perhaps, as I took my first bite of animal in twenty-six years, but there wasn't. The liver was, as I knew it would be, tough and rubbery because I'd totally overcooked it. Immediately, the taste put me back at school in the 1970s, hoovering up all the leftover liver because no other kid would eat it.

Taste is a strange thing because it has the ability to reconnect you with your past self from decades before quite viscerally and unexpectedly; it puts you, however fleetingly, intensely back in time, almost making you feel and think as you did – it's the nearest thing we've got to time travel. Momentarily, I was back in the school hall enjoying the liver all over again.

When I ate meat, right up to the moment I stopped, I was never a picky eater in any way at all. The only organ food I hadn't had as a kid was tripe. For some reason, mother told me I didn't like tripe despite the fact that I cannot recall ever being fed it. She and my dad ate it boiled in milk with onions. The bleached stomachs bobbing in an old aluminium pan of milk was a common sight. Let's face it, if you're going to have an animal killed, it's only fair that we eat all the edible bits – it's wasteful not to and, again, takes the piss out of the animal, much like those tasty kidneys, ironically enough.

So when I bit into the liver for the first time in twenty-six years the taste was alien in one sense because it was very obviously an animal but equally there was a familiarity that was oddly comforting in its reconnection with my childhood. That got me over the initial revulsion at the strong 'animal' flavour; it was as though I remembered liking it and so after a few bites it wasn't so shocking at all, indeed, though tough, it was lovely and as Masterchef's Gregg Wallace would say 'delicious, deep, rich iron'.

It was good to pop my meat cherry with liver. Perhaps

it was like deciding to take drugs and starting with crack cocaine. There's nothing polite or clean about it. It's a bloody organ from a dead thing. I knew that if I could handle it and cook it, I could handle and cook any meat.

And I could.

Because ultimately, though I was a bit freaked out by it, underneath that surface response lay the unsqueamish kid that used to shout 'show us the blood, Fred'. The sensitivity to the blood and the slaughter was just a veneer I'd chosen to apply back in 1984, but I now see that's exactly what it was, a veneer, an assumed attitude. Perhaps this is what all self-imposed morals are. There is nothing intrinsic about any morality we create; it is essentially a fabrication and they vary from generation to generation, culture to culture. What is heinous in one era is trivial in another. For example, when I was young, children born out of wedlock were a sinful disgrace, but now no one is bothered. I was sure I really believed in being a non-meat eater but when push came to shove, I didn't really. Underneath, I hadn't really changed. Eating it was, perhaps most oddly of all, like coming home. As though I'd been on a long trip abroad and after twenty-six years returned to where I started. I liked that. It surprised me and I felt good about it.

What I didn't know until later was that liver, along with being excellent protein, rich in iron and lots of vitamins and minerals, is also loaded with tryptofan, a chemical that essentially makes you feel a bit sleepy and nice and which has been reported as being a good anti-depressant. So 'Eat liver, Be happy' might be a good slogan.

And I ate the whole plate easily. Perhaps surprisingly easily. Dawn, not quite ready for the bloody horror of liver, had prepared a burger from minced beef and onion, ate all hers too, though, again, it was overcooked out of fear of bloody meat. We looked at each other afterwards. Both knowing each other had, within the limitations of the bad cooking, enjoyed it.

'Do you feel guilty?' she asked.

I sat for a moment and reflected, looking around our kitchen. Surprisingly, no, no I didn't feel anything. You can't fake such feelings. I had thought I might but I didn't really feel anything except relief that it was over, at least for a few hours. The handling and preparation of the meat had been more scary than the eating of it.

By 6pm it was time to eat again and we'd agreed to have a rib-eye steak each.

Now a bit more calm and having had plenty of time to research how to cook it, we went into the kitchen together. I seasoned the steaks with lots of black pepper and sea salt, heated a frying pan with some olive oil until it was very hot and fried the steaks. I was much less intimidated now.

It was hard to know how long to cook it for, after all we didn't have any idea how we liked our steaks. It wasn't a question I'd ever had to answer before. When we dined out at the Berni Inn and had T-bone steak it was always ordered well done. Indeed, looking back, every single cut of meat I had as a kid was well done to the point of being bone dry.

The idea that steak might be eaten when there was any red blood leaking from it was a total anathema to my mam and dad. It would have been regarded as simply wrong, as wrong as eating dogs. And not just wrong but dangerous. We were told you could get worms from undercooked meat. This may well have been true in the days before refrigeration, I suppose, and so the instinct was still to cook and cook and cook all meat. Raw was bad.

I had bought and cooked steaks with my own money on a couple of occasions in the summer before leaving home for college in order to impress girls, and impress them it surprisingly did, despite them also being cooked to oblivion. Come and enjoy my meat darling, is a chat up line I wish I'd used but, of course, never did.

So it's not surprising that as the steaks fried in the pan I somehow plugged back in to my 17-year-old self mindset and overcooked it. However, this was a top notch steak, the like of which I'd never had as a kid. We sat down to eat. I cut a piece of meat. The knife passed through it easily and smoothly.

As I bit into it and the flavour washed over my taste buds, I was amazed. A tingle shot down my spine. The rich meaty juiciness was mind blowing; like nothing I had ever tasted in my life. While the liver was familiar to me, this kind of steak was not. The times I'd had steak they didn't taste like this. My memory was a pale imitation of this experience.

This was organically reared and grass-finished. It was deep in flavour and had an iron-like liverish quality to it. After that first delicious mouthful, something remarkable happened to me. I tore into the rest of the meat hungrily, keen for another taste of the meat. I found myself even enjoying cutting the meat with my knife. It was exciting. I started laughing out loud as I found myself hungrily devouring the steak.

This was a raw, basic and quite shocking primal response. It was quite the weirdest I've ever felt when not on drugs. I couldn't speak while eating it, I just kept grunting like a beast as each juicy piece was chewed and swallowed. 'Oh fuck,' I kept saying like I was in the throes of some kind of orgasm.

The whole focus of my reality was that steak. It was all-encompassing. Dawn, who enjoyed hers too but perhaps not so viscerally, sat looking on at me with amusement. She later commented that I was actually hunched over the plate like I was protecting the meat from a competitor.

I've since reflected on this moment at length. I firmly believe it was one of the most profound of my life. In the few minutes it took me to eat that rib-eye, I was changed. That first mouthful, the way it tasted and the way it made me feel emotionally, was too genuinely profound to ignore. As I put my knife and fork down, I knew immediately from my response that my body was trying to tell me something, trying to tell me that this was the right thing to eat. I had gorged on it, devouring the whole 300g of it quickly. I had never felt like this before. The degree of satisfaction and satiation I experienced wasn't like any meal I'd had as a vegetarian. This caught me utterly by surprise. Perhaps it's like having sex for twenty-six years without realising you haven't had an orgasm, then one day, whoo-hoo, you find out what you've been missing for so long.

Once I'd finished, I didn't feel full the way I would have felt full after a typical soya and carbohydrate veggie meal. Instead, I felt not hungry but content. This felt great; the difference between satiation and fullness was huge. In fact I realised I had never felt like this before as a veggie, I had just eaten until I was full as opposed to when I wasn't hungry any more, which is a very different experience.

After eating I felt elated. I felt very strongly that the steak was really good for me; that it suited me; that it was feeding me properly. I based this on nothing but how I felt eating it. It was an entirely new sensation and, I must reiterate, it was a profound one. It might sound poncey but this is the only way to explain it: eating meat suddenly didn't feel alien, it felt deeply, innately natural to me, like I should have been doing it all my life, and it made me wonder what the hell I had been eating for twenty-six years.

This wasn't a vague or nebulous feeling; it was a visceral, core response, as deep and basic as lust or the desire to breathe air. It was a response that shocked me to my core. I hadn't thought I'd feel like this at all. It hadn't occurred to me that eating meat would stir my soul in any way at all except perhaps through revulsion. I thought I'd have to persuade myself that I found the taste acceptable or that I'd just enjoy it like I had enjoyed soya burgers. I didn't have a frame of reference for how this food tasted and felt to eat.

Not to be too weird about it but I really felt some sort of sexual stirring as I ate it. A lust. I don't know, maybe it was awakening the wild animal in me, the primal self red in tooth and claw! I know that sounds downright odd but I report it as I experienced it. It was as though a new life force flooded into me.

Despite only having the steak and some broccoli, I wasn't hungry again that day, which was odd because I usually needed to eat later in the evening. I also noticed that I didn't have any bloating or any feeling of discomfort that I almost always had after eating. It was like night and day compared to my usual post-eating experience.

But, overwhelmingly, what surprised me the most was how eating the steak had made me feel physically. I had absolutely no anticipation of the sense of digestive contentment and satiated palate.

I was surprised to find myself, at the end of the day, looking forward to having more meat the following day. I was also surprised that I didn't feel bad about eating meat. I had expected to have some remorse about it after twenty-six years of abstinence but my body felt so different even after just a few hours that, as unlikely as I admit it sounds, I quite distinctly, quite consciously sensed that it was doing me good; that my body was telling me this was what it needed to work properly. It might sound fanciful but that is quite clearly how I felt.

The next morning when I woke up, considering I hadn't

eaten for fourteen hours, I was only slightly hungry. Remarkably I also had no urge to perform an outlandish expulsion. Weird. In fact, for the first time in literally years, I went to the toilet just once.

I felt different. I knew it from the moment I woke up. It was as though a violent sea was becalmed. It was so different, so profound, it almost scared me. It didn't feel like ... well, it didn't feel like me.

All day long I kept stopping and concentrating on how my body felt, expecting some of the old symptoms to return but they didn't. It felt so odd to feel what I would have to call normal. I could not imagine that it would continue.

That day I ate a decidedly un-vegan three-egg omelette for breakfast with some blueberries and wasn't hungry again for over four hours. This was remarkable. For lunch we set about roasting a topside of beef. A big joint of meat. I had no idea what a topside of beef was, or where it was from on the animal, but a bit of research guided us. We rubbed olive oil into it and then whacked it in a hot oven for fifteen minutes, then turned it down to 180 degrees to cook. We thought we'd try to cook it until it was medium, reading that really, to do meat until well done was the plebs' way and would not get the best out of the meat.

As it cooked, the smell of the meat roasting once again evoked childhood memories and filled the apartment with a delicious savoury aroma. We let it rest as advised and then cut into it. It was still pink in the middle and incredibly tender. Juices ran out of it onto the plate. We cut ourselves two thick slices. It was sweet and yet savoury, the outside caramelised and crunchy.

Again, it was so satisfying and delicious.

We had it cold with salad for tea and if anything it was even more tasty with a bit of mustard.

I felt great all day and into the evening, excited at what was happening to me.

I still had a lot to learn about how to prepare and cook meat but from those first couple of meals there was no doubt in my mind that I would continue to do so. No doubt whatsoever. I felt odd. I felt lighter and had a real spring in my step. I felt more alert and sharp. This didn't take a few days to happen, it happened right away.

In the days that followed, we made a list of other meats to try, quite consciously and deliberately working our way through it but with no idea in advance if the pleasure we'd got from the beef would be matched. You have to remember that exactly what all the various meats actually tasted like was something of a mystery to us. We thought we could sort of remember but were not sure if we really could. Twenty-six years is such a long time.

The next day it was time to experience the delights of lamb chops and we picked two quite small organic chops with a thick layer of fat on them. I had never cooked a lamb chop in my life or if I had, I couldn't recall it. Once again here was something that looked like it had been cut out of an animal. There was no mistaking it – it had a bone sticking out of it!

As I put them into the frying pan with a teaspoon of duck fat, I was amazed at how much fat they started to render. Using a new pair of tongs and after a few minutes of cooking on either side, I stood the chops on their fatty edges and browned the fat until it was crispy.

The whole apartment smelled of hot, fatty lamb – an unusual and very distinctive smell. In fact the whole place had already started to smell differently. Instead of the odour of tomatoes, garlic and herbs – the holy trinity behind so much vegetarian cooking – the scent of roasting meats and fat now clung to the kitchen walls.

Again we had no idea how we liked lamb – pink or otherwise. As a kid pink lamb would have been considered raw and thus inedible but Delia Smith said that it was virtually impossible to overcook lamb as it was so fatty and juicy. So we fried the chops for eight minutes on each side until golden brown.

I looked at the two chops on my plate, glistening with fat and steaming hot.

At first I tried to cut the meat from the chop with a knife and fork but quickly realised this was a pointlessly genteel exercise. So instead, I picked it up by the bone and started gnawing on it like a dog, scraping my teeth down to remove all the sweet, tender meat. I was astonished at how sweet and delicate it was. It was fantastic. Soft, juicy, fatty and luscious. To my new palate it tasted really luxurious.

Then I bit into the fat. The outer layer was crispy and salty; inside it was soft and creamy. To say it was a taste sensation is to understate just how revolutionary it was in my mouth. While you might be able to make an approximation of meat using processed soya, there is simply no vegetarian approximation of a slab of lamb chop fat.

It was greasy and succulent. The idea that if you were to be a 'healthy' eater you would discard all this tasty fat fearing it would clog your arteries seems not just a terrible waste but would also transform the experience into a much less fulfilling one. Add to that the fact that there is much nutrition in the fat as long as the meat is grass-fed and I already began to see some of the madness at the heart of modern low-fat food culture.

It was just two small chops but they were a complete meal, satisfying in every way, and they became an early favourite for us. Once again the primal aspect of picking up and eating a piece of meat on the bone was really very satisfying and exciting.

I liked the 'uncivilised' aspect of it: eating with my hands, perhaps like our ancestors would have, tearing at the meat with my teeth instead of politely using a knife and fork. That really appealed to me. It might be a commonplace thing to do for most people but for me it was quite the opposite. It felt as though I was revelling in the animal; intimate with it, almost.

I sat back after eating them with grease running down my chin, once again laughing at the pleasure such small things had given me. I toasted the lamb that had laid down its life for me.

Later we ordered some larger chops from a superb company near Lanark called Damn Delicious. I usually buy my steaks from them. They're not certified organic but they feed all their sheep and cattle on grass only and in the winter on kale. They don't get fed any grain at all and no antibiotics or anything else like that are used. In some ways it is superior to organic because organic doesn't require grass-feeding. Their steaks are magnificent and their Texel sheep chops equally so.

The Texel is a big chunky sheep and the chops likewise. You can hold one in one hand and tear at it like a caveman! The meat is robust and savoury; the flavour delivered to your taste buds by the river of fat it renders. However when it came to fat, our next meat adventure had almost none at all: wild venison.

Venison is often sold to us as a so-called healthy meat because it's low in fat. This, I now believe is utter nonsense because animal's fat is very, very good for most of us and certainly for me. However, regardless of our cynicism for 'healthy' meat we bought some anyway. Neither of us had ever eaten venison, it being far too exotic and rare for us as kids.

I simply don't believe any butchers sold venison when I

was growing up, so we had no idea even what it might look like. As it turned out, it was a dark purple.

These were wild Scottish venison steaks. I was surprised at how dense the meat was and how much extra cooking it took over and above its beef counterpart. I was starting to learn that it is the responsiveness of the meat to your touch that tells you how rare or cooked it is. The firmer and less springy it is the more it's cooked. So if it's very soft, it's still very rare. I only realised this after I had cooked these steaks for as long as I'd cooked the rib eyes but found them still very rare and bloody. I put them back in the pan for another few minutes.

I caramelised all sides of these two thick cuts in butter and olive oil after seasoning with lots of black pepper and sea salt, enjoying picking them up with the tongs and frying them on their sides. Playing like this with the meat seemed all part of the fun somehow.

Once they felt like they were almost firm, I took them out and let them rest for five minutes while I made a jus in the frying pan by simply adding a little water and scraping all the burnt bits of meat off the pan. I added a splash of cream to it along with a small sprinkle of thyme. This made a herby, rich, savoury sauce. Not much, just a tablespoon or so, but was fantastic served over the steak with some buttered broccoli.

People say venison is 'gamey'. I don't really know what this means but it doesn't sound good. It's certainly often used in a negative context. Gamey sounds like it should be a bit off, but in fact we loved the venison. It was a dense, rich meat; deep in flavour and really substantial. Because there's no fat on it the creamy, fatty, buttery sauce really brought out the flavour of the meat and lots of black pepper really enhanced the experience.

Perhaps because of our upbringing, this felt like very grown up meat; quite sophisticated really and quite expensive too. We thoroughly enjoyed it.

So we ticked off venison and moved on to chicken. Dawn prepared the first roast chicken I'd had for the best part of three decades. She rubbed organic butter, garlic, chilli powder and salt into the organic, free-range, pasture-fed bird and roasted her in a hot oven until the skin was crispy.

As a kid, I was only given the breast meat, certainly never the skin. I don't know why, I seem to recall being told I didn't like it. As the bird roasted, the whole apartment smelled fantastically of roast chicken and was hot as. As Dawn pulled it out the oven, I stuck a thermometer into the most dense part of the bird and watched as the needle climbed quickly to the 'poultry' mark. As I pulled it out, a river of clear juices ran from the puncture wound. It was perfectly cooked and still moist.

Dawn carved off a leg and served it up on a plate for me. After the chop experience I immediately picked it up, even though it was almost too hot to hold I couldn't wait, and bit into it with gusto.

Sinking your teeth into a chicken leg is quite profoundly not a vegetarian experience. You are aware of your teeth penetrating the skin and tearing at the flesh of what is very obviously the limb of an animal. This no longer bothered me in the slightest, quite the reverse. It seemed to enhance the experience.

The skin was crispy, salty, hot and spicy, and utterly orgasmic. I tore into the tender leg meat, my lips on fire from the chilli. It was so juicy and savoury, the meat juices washing across my taste buds. I was soon gnawing on the bone, picking off every last scrap of meat with my teeth until the leg was clean except for a couple of bits of gristle. My hands were coated in melted butter, chicken fat and chilli running past my wrists and down my arms.

This was a full, physical experience and I bloody well loved it. In contrast to my previous diet, it was such a bigger, more gutsy, visceral experience; more instinctive, more exciting. It engaged all my senses in a way that eating, say, a Quorn fillet just didn't. As odd as it might sound, it was more life-affirming – except for the chicken, of course!

Pheasant followed on from chicken; a game bird but to me tasted just like chicken. Delicious served with some sage butter.

Soon we were tucking into all manner of charcuterie, enjoying bacon and ham especially. The last thing we really got into was pork loin and pork chops. I kept overcooking them, largely because the instructions on Waitrose packages overstate the cooking time by about 50 per cent. Their pork, though organic, was rather lacking in flavour. However, once we ordered some from Laverstoke Park (which is where we order much of our meat from) it was a different matter. Their pork is in a different class altogether. Again, because it is grown for flavour the pigs are fattier, the meat sweet and tender and fantastic served with a spicy chilli and apple sauce.

As we ploughed our way through the whole menu of animal foods, I found myself loving each and every one of them with just a single exception: fish.

Fish are often thought of as different to meat by those who like to get the supposed kudos of being vegetarian but who still want to eat our piscine friends. Maybe they seem less 'animal' and perhaps less sentient.

I hadn't really eaten much fish as a kid outside of battered cod or haddock, insane really as I was born in Hull, a huge port so dedicated to the fish industry. In the early 1960s when it was about to rain, it always smelled of fish as the wind swepped in off the sea.

I really should have been eating it since an early age and I can't understand why it was such a small part of our diet as kids. It's a strange thing that Britain, despite being surrounded by water, really has no love affair with our piscine friends in some regions and actively rejects many tasty varieties as not edible. Go to the west coast of Scotland and you'll see trawlers catching huge amounts of langoustine, almost all of which will be shipped off to the continent because no one wants to eat it in the UK. Plenty of fish and shellfish caught in British waters have no market in the UK. For an island we seem very conservative when it comes to fish consumption, or at least until a TV chef such as Hugh Fearnley-Whittingstall encourages us to try something different. Half of the fish we eat in the UK is cod, salmon or tuna. As kids we never saw any fish apart from cod, plaice or haddock ... and we lived in Hull, one of the biggest fish ports in Britain at the time!

So because of this lack of fish history outside of the chip shop, I had no strong childhood recollections to plug into when it came to eating it as part of my new carnivore life-style. We hadn't even eaten it when living on the Black Isle in our last carnivorous year, though Dawn was able to cook a magnificent fish pie when the mood took her. Indeed, in the first year we lived together, she cooked a fish pie the like of which I'd never experienced. So good it still stands out in my memory. Her dad was also a big fisherman so she'd grown up eating lots and lots of fish. Consequently, she had no trouble reconnecting with that and wasn't in any way intimidated by eating fish. But I was.

I actually had to learn to have a palate for fish. There's nothing like fish is there? It doesn't taste like anything else and it does taste, well, fishy, and when you're not used to fishy it really isn't a good thing.

So I got around this by starting my fish adventures with non-fish-tasting fish such a kippers. We picked up some Craster kipper fillets and, man, they were superb. Smoky, rich and meaty without any fishy aspect that I could discern. From there I went onto non-fish-tasting fish such as cod. I had swordfish, which was lovely, though apparently somewhat naughty on the sustainable fish scale.

I had my first ever tuna steak and loved it. I'd managed to go my whole life without eating a tuna steak and when I tasted it for the first time on a camping trip prepared over a BBQ I was amazed at how delicious it was. All these experiences just thrilled me; all these new taste sensations were simply life-affirming and exciting.

So having enjoyed these very much, one day, a couple of months into eating fish, I told myself not to be so stupid and to relax about the fishy flavour of such things as mackerel, salmon and sardines and enjoy them.

I was just reacting negatively for no reason at all; some of the best restaurants served these fish and people loved them. There was simply no reason not to be one of them. It was just the unfamiliarity of it that was proving to be a psychological hurdle.

Letting yourself consciously enjoy something is a strange thing to say but once I felt it was an unjustified inhibition and had given permission to myself to like them, somehow I just did. This was especially the case with salmon, which I'd flinched away from initially. One day I lightly steamed a salmon fillet, dressed it in lemon juice and olive oil, seasoned it well and found it delicious.

Looking back on it now, this kind of thinking was all part of the mindset I'd developed to get me through this massive change in diet: to think positively about it and not to be afraid or be negative or fussy. So I learned to love fish and will now eat anything that you might find in the water, except perhaps a cross-Channel swimmer.

I decided to embrace change and not be conservative. This positivity comes quite naturally to me – I am one of life's optimists – but it was endorsed and enhanced by my radically improved health. Even though meat and fish were alien to me, the fact that I was feeling so changed and so good meant I quickly saw the adventure as a leap into a brighter future.

Within a few weeks of eating that first steak I was enjoying every conceivable animal product, feasting on it after twenty-six years of deprivation. Did I feel guilty? Did I ask myself rhetorical questions? Did I bollocks. I felt so brilliant, so strong, so damn healthy and free of all my old symptoms that I would have been an idiot to think it was anything except very, very good for me. All my old vegetarian principles were thrown to the wind and I embarked on a whole new, healthy way of life. Get in.

So how exactly did this new old-fashioned, meaty, fatty, fishy and creamy diet affect me? In short, in every way possible. It's now eighteen months since I quit eating meat and so many changes have occurred.

My IBS vanished immediately and has not returned, not even once for old times' sake. I get no bloating, no upset bowels, no stomach pains. It now all works normally and regularly as I remember it doing before I stopped eating meat. All those years of suffering are now a thing of the past. Wow. Mind blowing. I thought I was stuck with it forever. Even today, I am still amazed by this.

I've also lost a lot of body fat. I'd gone into eating meat weighing twelve and a half stone, having put on twenty-five pounds after easing up on the starvation diet. Within a couple of months I had dropped a stone in weight, all of which must have been fat, taking me from 23 per cent to 15 per cent body fat.

At the same time I began to put muscle on from my thrice-weekly gym visits. I became broader of shoulder and more narrow at the waist even though I wasn't working any harder than previously. This does not make me some kind of freaky muscle-bound hulk. When it came to muscle, I was coming from a very low base, a low base of virtually no muscle at all. If I got a mosquito bite on my bicep it would have instantly doubled the size of it. I was not about to subscribe to Beef Cake magazine, a popular read at our gym with the inflated blokes who do body building. Beef. Cake. It's not a good cake, the beef cake is it? But it was good to be stronger.

I have not had a single headache and I used to suffer from headaches all the time. Not to have had a headache in eighteen months is quite amazing. This isn't just a coincidence.

I have much more energy than previously. It's an imprecise and nebulous thing, energy, but in general it has meant that I've lost the long afternoon snoozes, been able to do more and more physical work without getting tired, am less tired after long walks, more lively in the mornings and just generally more robust.

In these last eighteen months I've not had a cold or even a sore throat. Not a sniffle. Not even after trips to London and being exposed to the haze of human bacteria that passes for air on the Underground.

I've slept so much better and wake up properly rested.

My mood has been remorselessly good. This has simply never been the case before. Not ever. It has not been an easy year at all. The recession has significantly impacted on our business and we've had to work hard to get through it all. On top of that, Dawn's physical and emotional health has been challenging to deal with but I have remained strong and able to cope. I have felt more able than normal to deal with the stress of life.

I'm not talking about being hyper or manically happy. It's not that extreme. It's just about feeling on an even keel most of the time, not getting aggravated, annoyed or uptight at trivial things, keeping things in perspective. Not going ballistic when things go wrong, not being so emotionally volatile. I've described it to friends as feeling as though my feet are more firmly set on the ground. More centred.

My eyesight is so improved that I no longer use my glasses for reading. This happened within three or four months of the new diet. While not 20/20 it is so much better than it used to be and I feel it is still improving.

My libido, virtually in retirement for the previous few years, has returned to its 21-year-old, thrusting level and not just that: somehow, probably due to better blood flow and less body fat, you're looking at a man who is harder and thicker than ever! Of all the changes to me, this is, of course, the least important at my age, unless I'm going to suddenly give the gigolo trade a go. It's thirty years too late to impress Dawn, who has been suitably unmoved by this turn of events. Largely irrelevant it may be but it does at least make me feel that I'm still vital in some way and not an increasingly shrivelled, flaccid old man. These things are important to your psyche.

We climbed our second Munro and took up camping again, something we hadn't done since 1981, enjoying an especially memorable long weekend on Mull in glorious sunshine. In August 2010, I reviewed over fifty shows at the Edinburgh Festival for *The Mirror*, a mammoth feat of endurance. I was writing three pieces a week for Football365.com and running DJTees seven days a week – all on top of starting to write *The Meat Fix*.

Effectively, I've been doing three jobs concurrently. So in this context, keeping stress-free, relaxed and in good humour seems even more surprising. I've had plenty of excuses to have a meltdown from time to time but I just haven't felt the urge to do so. It is as though my biochemistry has been totally changed. It's like living inside a different body with different emotional responses.

Then we moved house – 380 miles south from Edinburgh to rural Norfolk. We've moved around a lot over the years, but this one was the smoothest, least stressful ever. Or at least it seemed that way. We both took it in our stride even though we were moving from the centre of a capital city to an old thatched farmhouse in the Norfolk Broads. This more even, calm emotional response has been entirely typical since changing my diet.

The contrast to my previous decrepitude was like night and day. The quality of my life on every level, both physically and emotionally, improved beyond all measure.

This whole process was a midlife reboot. All the old habits and routines established over twenty-six years of being a high-carb, low-fat, healthy-eating vegetarian have vanished, and I've had to create something entirely new and different. I'd recommend it for this reason alone. It's so refreshing to change the habits you've got into a rut with, to take a few steps into a new culture and challenge everything you've become accustomed to. Change can be frightening but it's also very energising and exciting.

I was amazed and thrilled but also bloody angry. Angry at myself for not making the change sooner and for just getting in such a mental and moral rut over what I ate. But furious also at all those years of misinformation from doctors and from the health authorities and governments. The better I felt, the more my indignation rose.

This old-fashioned diet, full of lots of the foods that we're told are bad for us, full of saturated fat and cholesterol, had fixed me.

So I wanted to know how all this had happened and I set about finding out. What I discovered shocked me to my core. I had thought I might be writing about what it was like to surrender vegetarianism after so long but no, that didn't seem important now.

I realised that everything that I thought I knew about healthy eating was wrong. Everything most of us know about healthy eating is wrong. The healthy eating guidelines have not made us healthy, quite the opposite: they made me and have made many others very sick. We have record levels of obesity, Type 2 diabetes, digestive problems, depression, food intolerances and allergies. These conditions have been blamed on us, on our bad habits and greed and not the healthy eating advice, which in turn has been elevated to an almost holy status.

How did this happen? How did I get so conned, how did I get stuck in such a rut? I had to find out. To do so I went over to the dark side, to the world of alternative healthy eating research and theory. It was a hell of a journey. A real eye-opener. Quite rock 'n' roll and anti-establishment and not at all what the doctor ordered. Challenging, sometimes funny, sometimes hard to understand and yet ultimately rewarding. Like Lennon said, quite possibly from inside a large bag, 'All I want is some truth, just gimme some truth.'

EVERYTHING YOU
KNOW IS WRONG

We pulled into Joshua Tree in a car that was as big as a buffalo, a brilliantly monstrous mobile metal warehouse that had just eaten up the infinite hot, hot, hot summer miles of Nevada and Californian desert.

Joshua Tree is a small, sprawling town high in the Mojave Desert. Nearly 3,000 feet up, of the 7,000 people who live there, New-Agers, spacers, freaks and other seekers of better living through chemistry are well represented.

While this might be a reason for most people to give the place a wide berth, as a veggie traveller the opposite was the case. It was an obvious place to pull in and get something to eat from the local hippy purveyor of veggie comestibles.

We pulled off 29 Palms Highway onto a rough piece of land. A cloud of dust billowed up and over the buffalo-sized car only to be caught on the hot desert crosswinds, swept across the road, up and off into the distance, gone like a fleeting notion.

I got out of the metal buffalo, put on my Ray-Bans and stood looking out across the widescreen grandeur of the Mojave, my hair streaming out sideways in the hot wind, the burning late afternoon sun casting a vicious black shadow across the crumbling concrete road. It felt like a western epic. Here we were, two insignificant humans in a big ancient desert, a tiny part of some seriously big nature.

As I took the scene in, a big, grizzled, hairy guy, who looked like a bear that had recently rampaged through a Levi's store, jumped into an old pick-up truck, started her up, threw the tail end out and accelerated past where we were parked. As he passed me, he leaned out the window and threw me a peace sign. Instinctively, I responded with a Spock-style 'live long and prosper' hand sign. I figured it's what you'd do in a place like this. He was probably an alien.

He'd just collected his order at our destination, The Crossroads Café. A funky, ramshackle wooden shed of a café full of people who didn't look like most of America. We went in and ordered a seitan burger – whaddya mean, what's a seitan burger? It's made from wheat gluten and is an old Chinese and Japanese food. Yes it is.

While we waited for the food I took a look at the notice board. It was a cornucopia of alternative lifestyle services. Homeopathy for dogs, tarot readings, aura vibration or how would you like someone to come around to your house and perform a shamani ritual? Call Ayla. How about some craniosacral therapy, reflexology, shiatsu, hot stones or rain drop therapy? All available in Joshua Tree. And if that's not enough, why not be entertained, if that is the right word, by The Kirtaniya, who are, evidently, 'a neo-bhakti revolution' whose gig is chanting Hare Krishna and the names of other gods.

Far out, cosmic and solid.

I collected the food from a man who had a spider's web painted in henna on half of his face and his beard plaited into a ponytail, held in place with a black and white yin and yang bead. Yeah, of course. It was hard not to love the place. Part freak show, part circus, part café.

After collecting the food, I pushed open the door to go back out into the white light and white heat of the desert summer afternoon. As I did so, a small notice caught my gaze. It was pinned to the wooden door and written in small, neat, rounded letters. It said:

That which is, isn't. That which isn't, is. You are always where it's at.

What was it? A Zen riddle, perhaps? A thought to ponder on as you make your way in the world? It has always stuck with me and often seemed very apposite. No more so than when researching much of this book because everything I discovered turned my previous understanding on its head.

Back in the late 1960s there was a countercultural troupe called The Firesign Theatre who released an album called *Everything You Know Is Wrong*. This was a common viewpoint among the hippy generation who had grown up to reject – at least for a couple of years – their materialistic upbringing and the careers which had been their well-planned destiny. Briefly in the late 1960s, the world turned upside down and everything that was supposed to be a positive thing – money, materialism, marriage and organised religion – became the exact opposite of what a happy, healthy life should be. Well this was my food equivalent.

The fact that a cure had always been so close, so within reach for so damn long made me angry. I beat myself up about it for a long time. Why had I been so stubborn for so long? Why hadn't I changed my diet earlier? Why hadn't I questioned it more? And why didn't the medical profession ever even hint at this solution? Why were so many doctors so helpless when faced with my bloated guts and runny bottom? Why did they and why did I get it so wrong for so long? I was bloody indignant.

That indignation only intensified when, after a little more than a week of research, I discovered exactly what had gone wrong and how the change in my diet had fixed it. I hadn't found it previously because I simply didn't look for info about my condition in relation to meat eating. But surely, a doctor or a specialist should have? Isn't that their job?

An excellent source of information was The Weston Price Foundation, which though USA-based has 'chapters' all over the world, including the UK. It is a non-profit, tax-exempt charity founded in 1999 to disseminate the research of nutrition pioneer Dr Weston Price and is dedicated to restoring 'nutrient-dense foods' to the human diet through education, research and activism. Its tag line is 'For Wise Traditions in Food, Farming and the Healing Arts'. Quite what the healing arts are, who knows, and yes, it sets my 'warning: this might be hippy bollocks' alarm off too. But for all that, I think they talk a lot of common sense. It is very much opposed to the use of soya, vegetable oils and other contrived modern foods and perfectly summed up what had happened to me over all those soya-munching years. Discussing the nature of soya as a foodstuff, they comment that processed soy foods are also rich in something called trypsin inhibitors, which hinder protein digestion. Trypsin is an enzyme that degrades protein as part of the digestive process. Anything which inhibits its proper working stops food being digested properly. Textured vegetable protein (TVP), soya milk and soy protein powders, are made by treating soybeans with high heat and various alkaline washes to extract the beans' fat content or to neutralise their potent enzyme inhibitors. These practices completely denature the beans' protein content, rendering it very hard to digest. Now, I ate processed soya every day – three, four, five or six times a day – for twenty-six years. Even when not eating TVP or tofu I was drinking soya milk in my tea.

It was because I could not properly digest the soya that partially digested protein molecules, instead of fully digested, made their way into the lower bowel where they caused digestive irritation, inflammation and putrefaction, and created all my IBS problems. As this went on, the levels of hydrochloric acid (HCI) in my stomach deteriorated.

With a low HCI level in my stomach, the large amounts of carbs I was eating just made matters worse, feeding all the bacteria and leftover proteins that sat undigested in my guts with their sweet, sweet sugars therefore causing the slapstick farting and painfully bloated stomach.

Unable to digest the food properly, my system, treating the food as a poison, rejected it altogether and got rid of it as quickly as possible, which explains the runny bottom and endless passing of semi-digested food. This became an unvirtuous circle of decline. While soya initially disrupted my digestive process, once it had been broken almost any food caused the same reaction, which is why all my food exclusion experiments didn't work. It was only eating meat that restored the correct level of acid in my stomach and allowed proper digestion. Essentially, my stomach got what it needed to operate properly as soon as I had stopped feeding the monster with soya and carbs and introduced proper protein. Not eating many carbs means there's not much sugar in my stomach and that in turn allowed my gut flora to be restored to its normal level.

A little bit more research revealed why I was so tired so much of the time. As a voracious consumer of nuts, seeds, beans, pulses, soya and wholegrains, my diet was very high in copper and because of the lack of animal protein, low in zinc. So what? Doesn't your body sort this kind of business out? Some researchers assign many symptoms to a copper/ zinc imbalance. The leading dude in this is a chap called L. Wilson MD who says:

> Copper is needed in the final steps of the Krebs energy cycle called the electron transport system. This is where most of our cellular energy is produced. Any problem here causes fatigue, depression and other imbalances related to low energy.

How cool does the Krebs energy cycle sound? Right out of a 1950s sci-fi comic book.

This may go some way to explaining some of my daily symptoms. He reckons that when copper becomes too high, negative traits begin to develop. These include feeling spacey, having racing thoughts, living in a dream world and naivety. Other qualities include childishness, excessive emotions, sentimentality, a tendency to depression, fearfulness, hidden anger and resentments, phobias, psychosis and violence. He has noted that artists, inventors and other high-copper types often live on the edge, in part due to their high copper level. Copper can function as a psychological defence mechanism. It causes one to detach slightly from reality. This provides relief from stress for the sensitive individual. This, reader, was my life.

While accepting that, in a fit of self-diagnosis, it's easy to assign any list of symptoms for any condition to your own condition, it's undeniable that my diet was heavy on copper and light on zinc and that this description is pretty much who I was for over twenty years.

Did anyone in the NHS ever mention this? What do you think? The trouble is, the modern 'healthy' diet with its emphasis on being light on animal protein and heavy on grains, starch and vegetable matter is also likely to be contributing to a copper/zinc imbalance in a way that more old-fashioned, meat-and-egg-centric diets simply wouldn't be. When I adopted this old-fashioned diet, it may explain why I developed such a marked improvement in energy.

The increased mental acuity can be attributed to the increase in the essential fatty acid, omega-3, found in wild fish and grass-fed meat, as well as a huge decrease in omega-6, found in all the soya and vegetable oils so dominant in my vegetarian diet. The reduction in carbs also meant my blood sugar levels were more stable. This then stabilised my energy and moods. On top of that, eating more fat slowed my digestion down and further evened out the blood sugar peaks and troughs, giving me a more even, calm and regular flow of energy. It also explains my improved sleep patterns.

Hurrah, clever me. It only took me my whole damn adult life to find this out.

The increased muscle bulk happened quickly because I was eating complete protein for the first time in twenty-six years. While many claim soya is a complete protein and others dispute this when it comes to being digested and absorbed, whether it is or not, there's simply no question that within three months of eating meat instead of soya I was considerably stronger and more muscular, and this process has continued ever since. So I'm not even interested in having an argument about how good or otherwise the protein I got from soya, seeds, nuts and legumes might be. You can say they're adequate if you want but in terms of how my body used it, meat beats it hands, hooves or trotters down.

Changing my mindset to challenge my low-fat, healthy veggie diet was the key. Until I accepted that I didn't do the right searches or look in the right places, I didn't and couldn't believe that everything I thought I knew about food and healthy eating was wrong.

I never wanted to be a doctor, other than a rock 'n' roll doctor, perhaps, but say hello to Dr Nic. Self-taught, with no diplomas, no degrees, no years at medical school but none-theless, with a couple of weeks of comprehensive research, I have managed, albeit in hindsight, to dissect and discern what has happened to me and why.

Despite medically qualified people being so stumped, so puzzled by it all, despite them getting things wrong and wrong again for years, it wasn't so hard to understand really. Once I got onto the trail, it all fell into place quite quickly.

None of this has ever been mentioned by any doctor or specialist I have seen nor, as far as I know, is any of it accepted as true, even in the absence of any other diagnosis. Not one element of it. There was never a suggestion that my healthy diet was the whole and sole cause of the problem – that would have been heresy. They want more people to eat like I ate, not fewer. This seems to have stopped them even think-ing for a moment that a low-fat, high-carb diet was crippling me. So if they were ignorant of all this, what else didn't they know? This was what sat up and hit me in the face after I got through all this.

Aside from the IBS, I had long thought all my other slow deteriorations of health had been merely part of the aging process. I was wrong. They were all because of my diet. My healthy, low-fat, wholegrain, cholesterol-free, vegetable-rich diet. Yes, I'll keep saying that because it's such a mantra that this diet is so good for you. Just look at all the healthy eating literature. None of it will tell you not to eat like this. Since I have dumped this diet, I've lost all those elements of degeneration. So who is right and who is wrong?

It was like putting a light on in a dark room. Even though

I had lost any faith in doctors to diagnose me, I still clung to the idea that my diet had been basically very healthy. On reflection, this was obviously ludicrous as I was ill. But I'd swallowed the orthodoxy whole. I believed it because it endorsed my life choices and, worse still, it made me feel superior. I was following the golden path, or so I thought.

Once I had thrown back the curtain on this assumption it all quickly fell apart as I discovered time and again reasons for both my illnesses and my new, improved condition.

However, all the sources of information that I used are all distinctly non-mainstream and their analysis is almost certainly not accepted or, more accurately, not even known about by your doctor. As you will already know, I couldn't give a toss what the medical establishment or the idiot nutritionist at a health centre think – their ignorance led to me suffering for so many years. However, it is undoubtedly true that this alternative world has its fair share of crazies, stupids and delusionals; so some would say, does the NHS.

It's full of people who assert opinion as though it's fact. Any view, no matter how extreme or downright surreal, is out there if you look hard enough. So when you're going in search of health and food truths you really have to bear that in mind.

You'll notice as soon as you delve into this world that whenever anyone is writing about health issues and diet, one of the first things critics want to know is what the writer's qualifications are to be making his or her analysis. In football parlance, you've got to put your medals on the table.

For many, those who are not medically qualified via a university are quacks, deluded, ignorant, malicious or profiteering – or all of the above. And of course many people are. If you want to believe that fairies are making the hair on your toes grow, then someone, somewhere, will offer proof that this is so.

The long and short of it is that you have to have your bullshit detector on when looking for medical and nutritional information. Of course you do. Only a fool would think otherwise. However, it's my view that the very same bullshit detector is also needed when entering the doctor's surgery

Just because they spent five years at university lighting each other's farts, does not mean they have much, or indeed any, clue whatsoever about what is making you ill, particularly when it's what we might broadly call a lifestyle illness. It's OK if you go in there with something hanging off or sticking out at an odd angle. They're good at spotting that. Anything that you can poke with a finger is easier to diagnose. But when it comes to diet-related problems, well that's all just a lot harder, especially in the allocated ten-minute time slot.

This is often said to be because most GPs have little or no training in nutrition, so you won't get any detailed or specialised advice from them. That would certainly be borne out by my experience. However, this doesn't mean that they recognise their limitations readily or that they'll be pleased at all the work you've done on your own. Quite the reverse in fact. When they say, 'Did you read that on the internet?' it will be said in a tone that suggests you have been to see the local witch doctor. I've seen doctors pout like sulky children when they hear you've been researching your own condition. I've seen them get snarky and short-tempered because you ask them questions and don't accept their word as an oracle of infinite truth.

Perhaps it's a bit galling for them really. There they were for decades, able to assert that Mrs Jones had Wobbly Flange

Syndrome or whatever with great medical authority without someone turning around and saying, hold on there bubba, that's not Wobbly Flange Syndrome; I think you'll find that's Hobbit-Induced-Gurgle-Honking and here's some research to prove it.

I'm sure there are exceptions to this generalisation. There must be doctors who know as much as there is to know about food and nutrition but I'd wager they are few and far between. That kind of detailed specific knowledge isn't your GP's gig is it? They're not called a General Practitioner for nothing. This seems to be where the problem lies. Yes, they can refer you to a specialist (who may also be useless, I know), but they can't if they know so little that they won't even consider food is the problem behind your condition. You can't prescribe a solution, even one administered by someone else, if you don't know it exists. It's my view that the first question a doctor should be asking when you present them with almost any condition is 'What are you eating?' If it's not directly related to that condition, it will be inseparable from how you recover from it. A badly fed body goes wrong. It doesn't work properly. You can't just ignore that. You can't just think food is some sort of peripheral influence on your body; it is the main influence.

Those who laugh at the quacks, loons and hypochondriacs need to wake up and realise that in many health centres there are also doctors with all the official qualifications but who are useless to some of their patients, especially when it comes to anything food or diet related beyond the obvious stuff such as 'It's probably not a good idea to be drinking turps Mr Nicholson and no, snorting bleach doesn't count as one of your five fruit and vegetables a day.'

Indeed, those who fall into the arms of the quacks mostly only do so because of the failure of 'conventional' medicine

– in other words, the dogma issued by those with the respectable qualifications. They are filling the void left by the inability of their GP to sort things out or because it is taking them so long to do so. Is it any wonder after such experiences people say, sod that, and go for self-diagnosis?

Dawn had a classic experience in this regard when she went to the ENT specialist because her sinuses were always blocked. The woman she saw was in her mid-twenties with huge fat buttocks who put me in mind of Kenny Everett doing his Rod Stewart impression way back when ... look it up on YouTube. Essentially, his arse inflates to enormous proportions. When medical people are radically out of shape it always worries you doesn't it?

It turned out she knew less than Dawn did about blocked sinuses. Dawn had asked the large buttocked woman, 'Do you think this could be hormonal rhinitis?' But she hadn't heard of hormonal rhinitis, even though it's so mainstream it's on the NHS website. And that was a 'specialist'. Useless.

Now, I'm sure there are better ones out there but how many and what are the chances you're going to get the good one? Quite small, I'd guess. You're forever playing a form of Russian roulette. Will you get the good one or the bullet? And you've waited for months for this brief interlude of mediocrity. Time fades away and nothing improves. You can't wait forever.

If this specialist had been a so-called quack, she would have attracted a stream of opprobrium and accusations of lack of learning for this performance, but she was protected from that criticism by the plywood door of her office in the bowels of an Edinburgh hospital.

Trouble is, the online debates around food and diet always go the same way. A self-appointed diet guru will recommend something and in response someone will post that they are a quack (the word quack is used a lot in such debates) because they have misunderstood or falsely reported the science they claim justifies their recommendations.

If the diet dude has got a PHD but it's in Maths not medicine and their only qualification is something from a college of nutrition which you can buy on the internet, this will further attract the quack accusation and consequent rubbishing of their ideas as bad science and little more than snake oil salesmanship.

It seems to me that critics who are understandably keen to spot bullshit when they see it are just as likely to be prone to believing notions, scientific interpretations and outright opinion that supports their own established world view as the wackos who believe evil pixies live in your stomach and cause all the problems.

However, they have one more arrow in their quiver (good word quiver, Sutherland Brothers & Quiver, not so good). They will sneer at the latest writer of a diet book because they're just 'selling a product' and so can't be trusted. They are tainted by the vast riches that the publishing world has to offer a writer. Unlike those hairy old professors in universities and research labs whom they seem to trust more.

However, research scientists need funding and take money from all sorts of interested groups that want them to come up with specific results. They can protest that this does not influence the result, maybe they do, maybe they don't but it's not as though money plays no part in the process.

The idea that there is no money, ego or a career wrapped up in scientific research is just naive and has been proven time and again. I totally understand that people want to knock down the latest fad diet and the theories that go with it – and fair enough if you want to do that – but one thing a few hours of research shows you is that there are so few hard and fast facts about food, diet and how it affects us that trying to take the intellectual high ground, whichever side you come from, never looks convincing. Even the most definitive statements tend to come with some caveats.

And let's not forget that 'official science' has delivered us a right bunch of old rubbish over the years and passed it off as hard fact. Drugs such as Thalidomide had previously been declared safe that were extremely harmful. Conditions and diseases are routinely falsely diagnosed and cures given that didn't and don't work.

They told us, unequivocally, that cholesterol in eggs would kill us. Then realised that was wrong. They said the same thing about too much salt and now that's disputed. They originally said trans-fats were healthier than animal fats – now they know they got that one wrong. Had non-medically qualified researchers argued they were wrong on those three issues at the time – and they did – they would have been decried as quacks. But they would have been right.

Given this, we'd be idiots to assume any proclamation to be the whole, absolute truth, no matter where it's from, no matter whether the team declaring it have academic qualifications or not, if they are from Harvard or from the College of Lunatics and Weirdos. None have a monopoly on the truth but some people on both sides want us to believe the good guys are all on their team.

This isn't to say that you believe anything you're told by anyone who has written a website or a book. So many diet gurus' work offers itself up as the definitive solution to whatever problem it is they're addressing – usually obesity and weight loss, which is where the big money is. Despite what all sides might tell you, it seems fairly obvious now that there is no definitive solution that applies to or suits every person. There are too many variables, too many differences born out of health, genetics and lifestyle which are constantly playing out against the shifting sands of your daily diet.

I guess the problem is a diet that says 'this might work but it might not' doesn't sell well. Nuanced messages, especially in the twenty-first century media, are not popular with publishers and media whereas simple black and white headlines are. Indeed, even when health studies report a nuanced message, it will get simplified by the media into a definitive statement it was probably never intended to be.

Thus diet books seem to feel obliged to have an almost evangelical approach to their subject. This in turn leads critics to point to those who have tried the diet to no effect and say, 'Well, it didn't work for them, therefore it's rubbish.'

It's too often all or nothing in this game.

So when you're an easily confused ex-stoner like me, who is just trying to find his way through life, have a good time and feel good, it's all too tempting to dump all sides into the bin and say, 'Feck the lot of youse' in the kind of belligerent Glaswegian accent that you might use if you lived in East Kilbride and your local off-licence had run out of Carly Special.

In the face of a bewildering amount of conflicting advice, we like to select our own medical advice to suit our own prejudices. It's much more fun.

If drinking wine every day is declared good for your health and we're wine drinkers, we think hurrah, I knew I was right all along and open a new bottle. If it's declared to be increasing your chance of getting cancer of some part of your body you didn't even know you had and couldn't find with your hand, you think, bollocks, my grandad drank like a fish and he never got that.

This is where most of us are today, I reckon. We want to know what's right and what's wrong but just don't trust anyone, no matter how well qualified or otherwise, to tell us the truth; or we rather suspect the current viewpoint is just another staging post on the road to the truth and will be overturned soon enough.

This is actually probably the most sensible approach: ignoring the bollocks which comes at us all the bloody time. Makes perfect sense. Tune it out like so much white noise. Maybe this is one reason why so many people have developed so many health issues caused by food: we've stopped even thinking about it and are just doing what the hell we want, drifting from one fad or fashion to another on a whim or a fancy or on a third-hand recommendation in search of something which makes us feel great, lose weight or gives us firm thighs, but never really finding it. It's understandable if so.

After eighteen months of research, I personally found that the most powerful information does not come from official papers about the effect of long chain fatty acids on your dangle-hosen gland, or whatever, it comes from personal experiences.

When you read that someone has achieved good health by following a specific regime, especially if they previously suffered from a condition or symptoms that you too are experiencing, it makes that regime have much more power to you. It might not work for us, we know we are all different, but then, it might. And that is about as much as we can hope to cling to when every side shouts so loudly that they in the right.

I have no qualifications in medicine or anything else food-related and I'm happy to admit it. I don't own a chain of health food stores, nor do I have a range of snack bars, diet powders, colon-cleaning potions or hats made out of quinoa flakes to sell you. I don't have a research grant to protect, a university to justify my job to or a pharmaceutical company rep trying to sell me drugs. This seems to make me different from almost everyone who has written about a specific food or lifestyle regime. Maybe I should develop some sort of supplement that helps you cope with all the bloody healthy eating advice that we get spoon-fed almost every day by the government and health professionals.

I only have my body, my mind and my experiences to inform me about how food affects my health – but we are all in that position though, aren't we? You've just got to make the best of it. If you're a proactive person and want to get well, we both know that hanging around for two months for your three-minute appointment with a specialist is likely to be a waste of time and take you no further forward, especially as the specialists really can't know any more than you can find out for yourself; and, in my experience at least, it is often a lot less.

So this is where you find yourself; torn between official advice, now quite redundant and the wild west of the non-mainstream world where people are wise, weird and wang-dang-doodle.

The problem is, everyone, be they a doctor at your local health centre who is exhausted after a day dealing with idiot people who don't understand that hitting yourself in the face with a brick might be the cause of their frequent nosebleeds, or the pearly-toothed American food guru weirdo who advocates a coffee enema every three hours as a cure for everything, they all dispense their information as though it is handed down from God. The absolute truth. So when you try their cure and it doesn't work, is it any wonder we get cynical about everything and everyone?

And this is before we get to the whole business of peer reviewing. As you'll know if you've ever read any criticism of anyone in the nutrition/diet movements, the demand from critics of any theory is always for their science to be peer reviewed.

It seems the holy grail for anyone critiquing any biological, medical, nutritional and dietary theories is peer reviewing.

In science this is the accepted method by which the potential veracity of well-researched theories is distinguished and separated from ordinary common or garden opinion and wild speculation.

The theory is if a selection of peers in similar fields review the work and declare it interesting and well done, then it can be published and be regarded to have some credibility.

If your work has not been peer reviewed, many will just dismiss it as worthless or at best just a piece of speculation or opinion.

While I can see the value of this to some degree, at least in theory, it is a very flawed system as history has surely proved. There are hundreds, if not thousands, of peer-reviewed pieces of work and research that went on to be proven as nonsense. It is far from an infallible system

As a layperson I'd have thought one of the problems is that every peer reviewer will have his or her preconceptions about how things should be done and if you don't do your work in a way they approve of they'll dismiss it. I also just don't trust any human to be that dispassionate about subjects which are close to their heart. We all get defensive and reactionary when our principles or long-held theories or beliefs are challenged, even if we know we shouldn't.

And another thing bothers me. Who is peer reviewing the peer reviews? Are they all of equal merit? What common standard is used to judge the efficacy of their work? It all seems a bit of a botched job to me. In theory it might be OK, but in practice, science, just like the arts, is every bit as subjected to the biases, whims and egos of those involved. The idea that it's all super-brainy people looking totally objectively and comprehensively at new research is to misunderstand human nature.

It might be the least bad of concepts for sifting the valid

research from the speculative and the loony, but it's not the cast iron system that those whose first instinct is to decry non-peer reviewed theories would have you believe.

And it seems I'm not alone in thinking this.

Richard Horton, the editor-in-chief of the The Lancet, Britain's primo medical journal said:

> The mistake, of course, is to have thought that peer review was any more than a crude means of discovering the acceptability - not the validity - of a new finding. Editors and scientists alike insist on the pivotal importance of peer review. We portray peer review to the public as a quasi-sacred process that helps to make science our most objective truth teller. But we know that the system of peer review is biased, unjust, unaccountable, incomplete, easily fixed, often insulting, usually ignorant, occasionally foolish, and frequently wrong.

It's worth bearing this in mind when you read comments on websites and blogs criticising any theories as not being peer reviewed and, thus, unreliable. Whether it's been peer reviewed seems less important; whether it's right or not is much more pertinent.

I accept you have to have some standards, some way of sifting the millions of pieces of research and recognising the brilliant from the bullshit. And I'm not saying it shouldn't be done, but all the same, just because a theory isn't peer reviewed doesn't make it wrong per se.

All that being said, there are some famous examples of plain wrong biology being passed off as though it's medical insight. Possibly the most notorious was Gillian McKeith, who as you might know was a TV nutritionist, or possibly a nutritionist on TV, or possibly just someone on TV. Anyway, she looked at people's poo in order to determine what was wrong with them – a neat if gross-out TV riff – even though it was usually self-evident that what was wrong with them was that they ate their body weight in chocolate and crisps every day.

Ben Goldacre, who runs the Bad Science website and writes for *The Guardian*, eviscerated her for the nature of her qualifications and what he considered her fundamentally flawed, bordering on fraudulent, ideas:

> She talks endlessly about chlorophyll, for example: how it's 'high in oxygen' and will 'oxygenate your blood' – but chloro-phyll will only make oxygen in the presence of light. It's dark in your intestines, and even if you stuck a searchlight up your bum to prove a point, you probably wouldn't absorb much oxygen in there, because you don't have gills in your gut. In fact, neither do fish. In fact, forgive me, but I don't think you really want oxygen up there, because methane fart gas mixed with oxygen is a potentially explosive combination.

This is just one example of his thorough savaging of McKeith to which she responded with quickly withdrawn legal threats. No point threatening to sue someone if they don't back down and then fail to do so when they are defiant.

The looking at poo-in-a jar TV gigs seems to have dried up for Gillian these days. The whole schtick was only ever going to have a limited appeal but then again, her company McKeith Research Ltd seems to be doing very well selling 'Personal Health Profiles' and all manner of supplements such as 'Organic Energy Powder', which does sound like a euphemism for cocaine, doesn't it?

Personally speaking she looks, what my gran would have called, 'not quite right upstairs'. And it certainly appears as though some of her biology is suspect and it does seem she has, at the very least, made the most out of her qualifications, some of which seem to have been available in return for a fee.

She says she's an 'internationally acclaimed holistic nutritionist' and who am I to say otherwise? Ben Goldacre's spat with her was all about the veracity of her ideas and the quality of her qualifications. This is quite typical of such clashes.

Clearly, passing yourself off as an authority on something even if you're not is a bit iffy but then again, what harm do people like her really do over and above the medical profession, other than give false hope, a trait all too common in mainstream medicine? Have they killed anyone? I'm sure we'd have heard if she had. It's not like she's getting someone hooked on tranquilisers is it, she's just telling people to eat more goji berries or pumpkin seeds or whatever.

This isn't to say that I agree with her. I've not even read that much of her stuff but it all seems to me pretty much like the old school hippy wholefood trip dressed up with a bit of science and you know where that got me, health-wise.

It just seems that it's so easy to vilify people such as her because of their profile and wealth but, frankly, people like her only have any success and any traction with the public at all because of conventional medicine's abject failure to address their health issues successfully.

People don't run into the arms of some strange woman on TV clutching a jam jar of their own poo before they go to their own GP, not even if she is wearing a very, very white coat. By the way what is it with a white coat that does that? Are you impressed by a white coat? No, me neither. So why do people who want to be thought of as science-y, doctor-ish types wear them? Why does it work? I'd be more inclined to believe a doctor if they wore a Van Halen T-shirt. At least you'd know they were into rock 'n' roll. People in suits make me nervous.

However, all that being said, you can feel suspicion or dislike for these self-styled nutritionists and diet gurus, and God knows there's no shortage of them, but if everyone's health and diet issues could be fixed at the local GP's surgery then no one would ever show interest in any alternative message; no one would take supplements or follow wacky diets.

The fact that people are so proactive that they go into their local health food shops, buy mineral supplements, packets of flaxseed and extracts of Horny Goat Weed is actually a good sign. At least they're trying to sort themselves out and take responsibility for their own well-being. Yes, we all get led up the garden path sometimes and end up buying some useless potion or product, but that is exactly what happens in a doctor's surgery too.

'Try this and if it doesn't work, come back and we'll try something else.' It's the doctor's mantra. We've all heard it. What it really means is, 'I have a range of things that I can prescribe but I don't know which one if any will work.' If this was said by an amateur or an alternative therapist they would be laughed at. But it seems OK in the doctor's surgery.

When you're not well and your doctors have been useless, all you can do in the face of the bewildering sandstorm of constantly fluctuating information advice and opinion – of which I fully realise this book is another tiny grain – is to use our own common sense to judge if the ideas, research and advice might be appropriate to your condition. It's still a very hard road to follow.

After all, what is common sense? I'm not sure if I've got any or maybe I'm full of it. How do you know? The things my mother and father thought were common sense were often absurd nonsense. Burnt toast makes your hair curly. Mother?

Are you sure? Is the Arab-Israeli war really caused by them 'eating all that garlic and chilli'?

One person's commonsense is another's howling lunacy. But all the same, you've got to try and weigh up the efficacy of all and any advice you can get.

So with all these factors in mind, put your stout trousers on, take hold of my slightly moist hand and let's follow that rabbit down that hole. Remember what it said on the door of the cafe in Joshua Tree – 'Everything that isn't, is. Everything that is, isn't.'

GREASY HEART

You can't eat anything these days; everything is bad for you. How come when we were kids, nothing was ever bad for you? Not even smoking was bad for you! Now every week there's a new report saying something else is now on the unhealthy-it-will-kill-you list; usually it's something they used to say was good for you. I don't believe any of them anymore. It's all bullshit. I don't believe any of these so-called experts know anything.

This was said to me by a friend last year and I had to sympathise. The amount of healthy eating stories in the media seem limitless and yet we don't seem any better informed as a result. Quite the reverse if anything.

I thought I had a good basic knowledge about food and what was healthy and what wasn't. Indeed, I considered myself smarter than the average bear about such matters. Or rather, I knew what I had been told was healthy food and what wasn't but by whom, well I couldn't actually say, specifically. Do you know how you came about your food knowledge? Do any of us?

Looking back, I seemed to have absorbed it by osmosis from hundreds of different sources over the years. When I stopped to think about it though, I had no idea of the truth of this learning. I didn't know on what research, if any, it was based. I didn't know who might have done such research or who paid for it. I did believe, however, that there was a fairly settled medical view on what was and wasn't healthy and I was also pretty sure that my wholegrain, zero-cholesterol and low-saturated fat diet was on the right side of the fence. If I had ever been in any doubt, doctors and health centre nutritionists had reaffirmed it. They couldn't all be wrong could they?

Well, yes. Pretty much. I was a walking, or rather, hobbling example of how destructive it can be, wasn't I?

Put simply, on one side there is the current default healthy eating advice: don't eat much fat (especially animal fat), use vegetable oils, don't eat much red meat or sugar, eat lots of fruit and vegetables and make sure a third of your plate is starch, made up of wholegrains, rice, pasta, bread and potatoes.

Everyone except the real window-lickers know this mantra now. It's been around for thirty years and, like me, you're bound to have absorbed some or all of it. Whether you've taken any notice is another matter of course. I hope you haven't.

However, I didn't realise that this was merely one side of the debate. There is another world, a more gothic world, the dark side if you will, which is the land of the alternative healthy eating theories. Almost all of the theories disagree with this conventional wisdom wholly or to a large degree. Indeed, they are almost all contemptuous of the advice given out and consider it not just wrong but actively harmful.

Yet there isn't some sort of anti-healthy eating advice rainbow coalition, no single unified voice, rather, lots of different shades of often similar opinion. Perhaps that's why no single powerful opposition to the official guidelines has emerged, especially since each one seems to loudly proclaim their way is the right way.

The most prevalent alternative orthodoxies, however, often fall under the general, if inaccurate, banner of 'low-carb' diets. That term in itself is somewhat misleading. Many are called low carb simply because they recommend eating less carbs than the typical modern diet, not because they are actually especially low in and of themselves.

There are many different strands to the low carb movement. Some are totally non-grain, others just anti-wheat, some very opposed to eating fructose in fruit, some more vegetable-orientated than others. For some it's part of a more primal, Palaeolithic, 'caveman' lifestyle and diet, a reconnection to more natural sustinence. Others focus on the balance between omega-3 and omega-6 fatty acids and controlling inflammation in your body. Whatever angle they're coming from, there is widespread agreement that we eat too many carbs, from grains, tubers, sugar and fruit and that this has impacted on the health of many people very negatively, leading to weight gain, diabetes, depression and all manner of other modern day conditions.

They are also largely pro-animal fat, pro-meat, pro-red meat and some are also in favour of pure dairy and raw milk. They usually consider the whole cholesterol issue – often called the lipid hypothesis – a myth and that the conventional healthy diet has made us sick. In short, they believe that it is the very healthy eating advice that we have been spoon-fed for thirty years that has been the root cause of all the health issues we see today.

The two sides could not be more diametrically opposed. Before my diet change, I had no idea that this was the case. I thought diets were all fads that were invented to sell books and that they came and went in and out of fashion. I didn't realise there was essentially a whole alternative universe of healthy eating theory; a bizarro world where almost everything we've been told is bad for us is actually good and almost everything we have been told is good is actually making us sick.

Obviously, once I learned this, I was attracted to it as a concept because by and large this was what had happened to me.

So let's take a look at some of the big issues when it comes to diet and let's start with the as-serious-as-a-heart-attack stuff. Saturated fat and cholesterol.

We're all obsessed with fat or rather we're obsessed with not eating fat. It drives so much marketing and so many products. 'Low fat', 'lower fat', 'zero fat', '% fat', 'high in polyunsaturates', 'low in saturated fat' etc. etc. is plastered over so many products. If we eat fat, we'll get fat. That's what we all consciously or subconsciously think. It's certainly the notion that the advertising plays to. However, I got fat eating a really low-fat diet. Well done me. Perhaps because the same word, fat, is used in two different contexts, fat in food and fat on our body, they have quite wrongly become conflated in our minds into one and the same thing.

Fat sounds bad, we've all got that message and we all feel instinctively that it'd be better for us if we didn't eat much fat at all. But if we're going to eat fat, most of us know we shouldn't eat much saturated fat. He's the bad boy. Polyunsaturated and monosaturated fats are the good guys, or less bad perhaps.

But do we know what saturated means or what it is? Do we bollocks. Let's look it up in a medical dictionary then. Apparently, 'saturated fatty acids have no double bonds between the individual carbon atoms of the fatty acid chain. That is, the chain of carbon atoms is fully "saturated" with hydrogen atoms.'

Errr. Yes. So we're all none the wiser then. Saturated fat actually sounds like very fatty fat to me. Like it's absolutely sodden with the stuff. Anyway, every doctor will tell you 'sat. fat' is the killer stuff which will give you a heart attack. So be afraid, be very afraid. Look at what the NHS Live Well leaflets and website says about this.

> Eating a diet that is high in saturated fat can raise the level of cholesterol in the blood. High cholesterol increases the risk of heart disease. Saturated fat is the kind of fat found in butter and lard, pies, cakes and biscuits, fatty cuts of meat, sausages and bacon, and cheese and cream. Most of us eat too much saturated fat –about 20 per cent more than the recommended maximum amount.

It lists all manner of ways to cut down your saturated fat intake including 'use reduced-fat spread instead of butter'.

Yes you are going to die if you eat butter. Better eat a factory-made contrived tub of gloop called low fat spread instead. They actually recommend this! Because obviously, the human race all died of heart attacks before the introduction of low-fat freakin' spread didn't it? What are you, stupid?

They tell you to read labels and not eat more than thirty grams of saturated fat per day. What happens if you eat twenty one day and forty the next, ten and then fifty, none and then sixty? No comment. Stop asking silly questions. Shut up and accept this truth.

It goes on and on about traffic light colourings on labels. Presumably red means death and green life. Grill sausages, eat low-fat yoghurt, less cheese, skimmed milk, dry-fry eggs (dry-fry bloody eggs, how the hell do you do that?), eat skinless chicken, blah blah blah. For God's sake. It's like being bossed around by an obnoxious dinner lady and is done in such a 'this is for your own good' tone that it makes you want to shout, slightly hysterically, 'Stop telling me what to do!'

It strikes me this is a very good way to turn a sane person into a gibbering wreck, paranoid about the nutrients in every food, fearing that everything is slowly killing you, as though every mouthful you take is another step towards the grave.

Listen, we're all bloody dying. Sadly, it's true. No one gets out alive. All we want to do is have a good time, feel happy and strong and complete our Jethro Tull record collection before it all goes black. And worrying if you've had more than 30g of saturated fat in a day seems as good a way as any of killing your enjoyment of life, let alone squinting at the label on every foodstuff you pick up and wondering if you can balance one with a lot of red marks on it against one with lots of green marks. This is no way to live. It's a form of insanity, the worry about which will do you more harm than the bloody food.

However, if you read closely, there's one piece of information that does make it through this fog of confusion, though it hardly announces itself loudly: it's not the saturated fat per se that will kill you. The danger it offers is that it can raise the level of cholesterol in the blood and it's that high cholesterol level that increases risk of heart disease.

Right, OK, so let's get to grips with this cholesterol stuff – we've all heard of it. What do we actually know about it? Cholesterol causes heart attacks. That's almost certainly the full extent of our knowledge about it. Where fat ends and cholesterol begins, well we don't really know do we? It all blurs into one big greasy dollop in our mind and in our arteries, though not our veins, for some bizarre reason.

It blocks those lovely pristine arteries doesn't it? Or is that the fat, or is it just the saturated fat? Who bloody knows? We probably think it all does. Something certainly clogs your arteries. One word has made it through the fog of confusion and that word is 'clog'. That'll clog your arteries. The word clog has become almost exclusively used in connection with the word arteries it seems. You'll see the expression 'artery-clogging foods' all the time in the press.

If you pour hot lard down a sink, when it cools it will harden and block it up. This is how we see what happens when we eat too much of that there cholesterol stuff, and fat too.

We've been warned about not eating a lot of cholesterol for thirty years now. That's what all the fuss about limiting how many eggs you ate was about, among many other dire warnings about drinking full-cream milk and cheese.

We're probably not sure how much too much is. We wouldn't even know how to measure it would we? We just know that too much is very, very bad. It's certainly how I viewed it for years. I had no idea that cholesterol is actually very important to the healthy working of the body or that most of my brain is made up of cholesterol. I thought it was a poison but, in fact, if you have no cholesterol in your body you will keel over and die. It's that important to us.

But nonetheless, the main message has got through. Cholesterol is bad, it'll kill you. Jokes are made about cholesterol-rich foods every day. Does that come with a defibrillator? All of that. Hilarious.

Ok, so far so good

But wait right there. Just when you think you might have got a handle on all of this, it turns out that all of this is, wait for it, yes, it's utter rubbish.

This is why.

The cholesterol we eat doesn't affect the amount in our blood. Who knew? Not me, not you I'd wager. For years the authorities said it did and they told us to be careful how much we ate didn't they? I didn't just dream that did I? No. It really happened.

Well they got it wrong. Oops.

Trouble is, many people, going back thirty years, always thought it was rubbish. Many in the medical community spoke out against it at the time it was established as 'truth'. However, through a long and complex mixture of effective lobbying, marketing and misinterpreted, hurried and selective science, it became established as a truth and one which was sent out as gospel to every doctor's surgery since the early 1980s.

So, being concerned about eating cholesterol is wrong. You've been worrying about nothing and I was wrongly feeling superior for not eating any as a vegan for all those years. Bugger.

Shall I state it again? The cholesterol you eat does not affect the amount of cholesterol in your blood.

Ancel Keys, the man whose much disputed studies in the 1950s led eventually, via a long and tortuous route, to the current state of play on cholesterol, said quite unequivocally, in 1997, 'There's no connection whatsoever between cholesterol in food and cholesterol in blood. And we've known that all along.'

Now, just three years after he said that my doctor told me that up to 30 per cent of the cholesterol in my blood came from my diet, which I knew simply couldn't have been true because I didn't eat any cholesterol. One hundred per cent of my cholesterol came from some other freakin' place. At the time I thought this was obviously nonsense but I was scared of the you're-going-to-die-of-a-heart-attack graph he showed me. That's why I took the drugs he gave me, officer.

But still to this day, most people think if you eat lots of cholesterol you are more likely to get a heart attack and it would seem to me that the health authorities are not doing much to shake this idea from our minds.

However, as we've seen from the NHS, the official healthy eating advice has shifted a little from this position on cholesterol consumption to being paranoid about saturated fat instead.

So despite previously being 100 per cent wrong in saying the cholesterol you eat contributes to your blood cholesterol level and despite them telling us not to eat more than a couple of eggs a week for fear of dropping dead from all that delicious cholesterol, they still want us to believe their latest advice, whatever it is, is correct. Well we're entitled to ask why the hell we should, I reckon, don't you? Had we questioned their advice on cholesterol they'd have assured us it was correct, just as they do now on saturated fat.

Don't worry though, having high cholesterol in your blood, even if you haven't eaten it, is still bad for us. In the UK any doctor will tell you that anything over a reading of five (five what? We don't know) is cause for concern. As happened in my case, they might present you with the heart attack vs cholesterol level graph which shows the increased likelihood of you having a heart attack or stroke due to this reading. It will scare you and you will then be put on the wonder drug statins.

These are the bestselling drugs in the world; naturally there is big money in preventing death, or at least in the assumption that you are preventing death because actually the original adverts for statins included a statement to the effect that they had not been proven to prevent heart attacks.

They haven't?! Hang on. What the feck am I taking them for then? Just in case, lad. Just in case seems to be the answer.

Imagine if you want to make an almost infeasible amount of money, what would you invent?

X-ray vision, obviously, and a way to stop parents bringing their children into the pub. But if it had to be something that is actually possible, how about a drug that would stop you from dying from the most common affliction today? Who wouldn't want that?

Heart attacks kill more people than anything, so why don't we invent a drug that will stop you from dying from a heart attack? Sounds ideal. Who wants a heart attack? No one, not unless you're a total pervert who enjoys indescribable chest pain, shortage of breath followed by a long period of blackness.

OK so a life-saving heart drug it is. Great. But hang on, here is an even better idea. We'll invent a drug that will keep you alive, but only if you take it every day. You can't get protection from it if you take it for a month or a year and then stop. It doesn't build up protection, not even if you take it for twenty-five years. If you stop after twenty-five years, you're at risk again immediately. Brilliant. It guarantees infinite sales for as long as there are people alive.

Marvellous. Now we're bound to make more money than God in Las Vegas on a winning streak. But hold on. What if someone does have a heart attack while on our drug? They'll sue us for every penny we've got. We don't want to risk that.

I know, our drug will lower the thing which some people say causes heart attacks: cholesterol. So it's not actually a heart-attack stopping drug, it's a cholesterol lowering drug. And you know what too much cholesterol will do to you don't you? Say no more. All we have to prove is that it lowers cholesterol for it to be sold as a de facto heart-attack prevention drug. If it turns out that cholesterol is nothing to do with heart attacks then we can't be held responsible for not preventing heart attacks. If our drug doesn't work then we'll just blame the people who said cholesterol was the problem.

Cool. We're sorted. It doesn't have to work all the time for everyone for us to sell it. I like it.

One statins manufactuer, Phizor, made $12.8bn in 2008 alone.

They do reduce your cholesterol for sure; I know this from my own experience, 40mg a day of Atorvastin made by Lipitor whose logo was strangely on the blood pressure equipment in my doctors surgery, halved my cholesterol level from 9.2 to 4.5. Have I had a heart attack? No? So they must work then! Err ... not necessarily. That rather depends on if you believe cholesterol levels have anything to do with cardiovascular disease, stroke, heart attacks or indeed anything at all in the first place.

Before I looked into this, I had no idea that there are doctors, researchers, scientists and nutritionists who simply don't accept cholesterol has any role in heart disease and have done much research into the matter. Indeed, there is a group called The International Network of Cholesterol Skeptics set up to promote this view. It might be tempting to think that this is a group of wack jobs who are trying to make a name for themselves. Well, if they are, they're not doing a very good job as I'd wager almost nobody has heard of them.

However, it is on the assumption that lower cholesterol means fewer heart attacks that statins have been declared a modern-day wonder drug. Cholesterol is at the nervously beating heart of so much healthy eating and health diagnosis.

You don't just take a course of statins for a week or two, you have to take them ... well ... forever ... or at least until some other non-cholesterol-related disease kills you. The trouble is, taking statins isn't without its dangers. I was warned about one of these, muscle pain. Stop taking it if bits of you start to hurt, was the advice. Oh and don't eat grapefruit. Eh? Why? Shut up and take the pill. Oh, OK. But the problems with statins don't stop with the odd twinge. There's a research organisation called The Marshall Protocol Knowledge Base which, among other things, collates the results of clinical trials and research on causes of chronic inflammation. It discovered, that:

> According to the reports from the statin trials, all of which have been sponsored by the drug companies, side effects are mild and rare, but under-reporting is prevalent. According to drug companies, muscular symptoms occur in less than 1 per cent of patients taking statins, however researchers independent of drug companies have found the frequency to be 64 per cent and 75 per cent.

In the impressively titled Incremental Decrease in Endpoints through Aggressive Lipid Lowering (IDEAL) trial, almost 90 per cent of participants in both groups had side effects, and in almost half of them they were recorded as serious.

So what side effects might you suffer from? It's not a pretty list. Lupus (I thought lupus meant you became a werewolf), pneumonia, dyspnea (pain while breathing), muscle pain, renal dysfunction, tendon complications, cognitive dysfunction. That's a pretty unpleasant list of adverse effects, most of which I think I've also suffered from after drinking that cheap white cider.

A 2008 survey of statin patients found that 75 per cent experienced cognitive dysfunction determined to be probably or definitely related to statin therapy. Of 143 patients who reported stopping statin therapy, 90 per cent reported improvement in cognitive problems, sometimes within days of statin discontinuation. In some patients, a diagnosis of dementia or Alzheimer's disease was reportedly reversed. Severity of cognitive problems were clearly related to statin potency.

Some say a large statin dose also increases your likelihood of getting Type 2 diabetes and even of having a stroke, which would be a bitter irony. If one thing doesn't get you, another will, it seems.

The Marshall Protocol research concluded that for adults aged between thirty and eighty years old, who already have occlusive vascular disease, statins confer, what they call, a total and cardiovascular mortality benefit. Which, in English, means fewer people die. This doesn't seem in doubt. However, 75 per cent of people who take statins are not in that category. If you are healthy there is marginal evidence that statins prevent heart attacks or strokes. One meta-analysis (that just means it rolls together lots of different bits of research) showed that in healthy patients there was only a 0.6 per cent reduction in mortality. In other words, physicians would need to treat between 100 and 450 patients with a statin for more than four years to prevent one death.

So there I would be taking this drug for maybe up to fifty more years. I would never know if it had prevented me having a heart attack, but because you're taking something, you probably assume it has even if you'd have been perfectly healthy anyway. The power of taking a pill is often said to be greater than the power of the actual pill. The placebo effect works and two placebo pills work better than one. Even if you're told it's a placebo. We are officially mental, aren't we?

Interestingly, these drugs become generic in 2012, therefore anyone can make them. The big money will then drop out of the market for those who hold the patent. I wouldn't mind betting far fewer statins then get prescribed as the big pharmaceutical companies' marketing departments move on to newer, more profitable drugs.

I was an early adopter of statins back in 2001; today, many feel they are over-prescribed, given to people who have not had a heart attack and have no history of heart disease. More traditionally we call these people h-e-a-l-t-h-y.

So that's where we all are. Loaded up on statins – seven million people in the UK alone are on them and we're all still scared of cholesterol, which it would seem, all things considered, is exactly where the pharmaceutical industry rather likes us as customers.

But if you'd been paying attention in the press, and many have which is why we're all so cynical about health and diet, in 2007 the UK 'health Czar' (if you're appointed a Czar you really should wear one of those big furry Russian hats at all times, I feel) was saying everyone should take statins. It was widely reported in the press in the summer of 2007 that statins cut the risk of heart attacks by 30 per cent even in healthy people and reduce the chances of death from all causes by 12 per cent. It was being suggested in some reports that everyone over fifty should be prescribed statins.

Oh wow. Groovy. Let's all hoover them up like they're M&Ms (or more accurately Treats, as my generation should still insist on calling them).

No. Hang on. Things have changed. Spool forward four years and there are more reports in the press and on TV saying something quite different. Look at what the BBC was saying in early 2011:

> Healthy people may derive no benefit from taking cholesterol-lowering statins, according to a review of previous studies. The report, published in The Cochrane Library, concluded that statins reduced death rates. But it said there was no evidence to justify their use in people at low risk of developing heart disease. The British Heart Foundation said the benefits of prescribing statins for those people was unclear.

Well OK, I was on statins for eight years but I'm not any more. I binned them eighteen months ago. Even for someone who had grown cynical about the science and motivations behind the pharmaceutical industry, it still took a bit of courage to throw them away.

Johnny's current health status: Not Fucking Dead Yet, Pal.

It was this paragraph from writer Andreas Moritz's book *Timeless Secrets of Health and Rejuvenation* (I know, I know, it does sound a bit New-Agey doesn't it, you can smell the camomile tea from here) that finally persuaded me I'd been prescribed something that was simply not needed and may well have made me ill:

> In an eight-year long heart study, researchers observed 10,000 people with high cholesterol levels. Half of them received a best-selling statin drug. The other half were simply told to eat a normal diet and get enough exercise. The results stunned the researchers. Although the statin drug did indeed lower serum cholesterol, this had no impact whatsoever on death rate, non-fatal heart attacks and fatal arterial disease. In other words, the statin-users had zero advantage over those who received no treatment at all … lowering cholesterol either through drugs or low-fat diets does not lower the risk of developing heart disease.

He goes on to say not only is there no connection between cholesterol levels and heart disease but also that reducing your saturated fat intake to reduce your cholesterol rate has no effect.

It is Mortiz's contention that all major European long-term cholesterol studies have confirmed that a low-fat diet does not reduce cholesterol levels by more than 4 per cent, in most cases merely 1–2 per cent, well within the margin for error and that, regardless, cholesterol levels naturally increase by 20 per cent in autumn and drop again during the wintertime. A more recent study from Denmark involving 20,000 men and women demonstrated that most heart disease patients have normal cholesterol levels.

'The bottom line is that cholesterol hasn't been proved a risk factor for anything,' says Mortiz.

However, the official advice is still totally unequivocal about the fact that 'high cholesterol increases the risk of heart disease'.

Had I bothered to find out at the time I was prescribed statins that there are very many people who believe the whole cholesterol issue has been a myth from the very start, largely drummed up by a variety of industries that benefit from everyone being cholesterol averse, namely the pharmaceutical industry, the vegetable shortening fat lobby and the soya industry. Because if we don't want to eat cholesterol, into whose arms do we fall? The greasy arms of the non-cholesterol vegetable oil industry, that's who. Into the soya protein industry's arms for our hit of protein without animal fat or cholesterol and to the drug companies who have made billions from cholesterol-lowering drugs.

It's not my aim to reiterate a lot of biological science in *The Meat Fix*. I lost interest in biology after we looked at a gerbil's reproductive organs, which seemed somewhat intrusive and abusive to the gerbil, not the least because the poor fella was dead and cut open from head tail. This was at school, of course. I don't cut open gerbils at home as some sort of weird hobby.

If you google 'cholesterol myth' you will find a lot of information about all these alternative theories on how cholesterol works in our bodies. It is, to say the least, open to question that cholesterol has any role in heart disease, at the very least for some people. As ever, I'm suspicious of generalisations because there are bound to be some people for some specific genetic or medical reason for whom it does work; but, without doubt, the commonly applied wisdom on cholesterol is not the whole story by a long way. This isn't just hocus pocus witchcraft. It's not part of some ropey old New Age-chakra massaging nonsense. These are serious people who have serious research to back up their theories. These can be summed up by quoting from *The Great Cholesterol Con* by Anthony Colp:

> Heart disease is not caused by saturated fat nor elevated blood cholesterol; people with low cholesterol levels live shorter lives; populations consuming high saturated fat diets often enjoy very low rates of heart disease; many dietary recommendations made by 'experts' to reduce heart disease have actually been shown in animal and human studies to increase heart disease, cancer, diabetes and obesity; the primary force behind the anti-cholesterol paradigm is not public health, but profit!

Once you read these books, it's not possible to believe unequivocally the advice from the NHS. But sit down opposite your doctor and say this and they will get narky almost immediately, start moving around uncomfortably in their chair, type 'troublemaker' onto your notes and then they will issue the party line once again. Along with a prescription for statins. In my experience, they are not likely to have read any of the books challenging the commonly accepted view of cholesterol. I have yet to meet a doctor who will even engage in debate on the matter. It is as though they believe it is a 100 per cent watertight argument. They will assert the orthodoxy as though there is no doubt about cholesterol and that their knowledge is absolute. This is why so many of us find doctors infuriating. They display too much certainty in matters which are undoubtedly in dispute. I know they don't want to look weak or stupid but to not address these issues at all and to pretend they don't exist or are little better than witchcraft or superstition demeans us all and undermines their own credibility.

As I write this, the cover story on *Time* magazine is 'What to Eat Now' written by some American talk show doctor fella called Dr Oz. (Is that his real name? Sounds more like the name a low-rent hypnotist would have.) On cholesterol he says, 'Dietary cholesterol is less important than we used to think and is irrelevant to some people who have good genes.'

So it's even reached the world of the TV doctors now. For over thirty years, we appear to have been sold either a lie or a best guess or a commercially driven notion about cholesterol. If it wasn't a lie it was what my grandad Fred would have called 'a massive dropped bollock, our John'. I think we should have an apology but will we get one? Will we bollocks. This is how the British Heart Foundation has weedled its way out of it in its Q & A section:

Q. I've heard that eating too many eggs can raise your cholesterol – how many can I eat?

A. For most people there is currently no limit on the number of eggs that you can eat in a week. However, because the recommendation has changed over the years, it's often a common source of confusion. In the past a restriction on eggs was recommended because we thought that foods high in cholesterol (including liver, kidneys and shellfish, as well as eggs) could have an impact on cholesterol levels in the body.

However, as research in this area has developed, so has our understanding of how foods that contain cholesterol affect people's heart health.

For most people, the amount of saturated fat they eat has much more of an impact on their cholesterol than eating foods that contain cholesterol, like eggs and shellfish. So unless you have been advised otherwise by your doctor or dietician, if you like eggs, they can be included as part of a balanced and varied diet.

Well, thanks for that. No mention that there always were scientists, doctors and researchers who said it was all rubbish and who were ignored. Whole industries grew up to service the low cholesterol food demands that arose due to this hypothesis. I remember seeing 'eggbeaters' for the first time in California twenty years ago. They were commonplace over there and had been since the late 1970s: merely a carton of egg white, with the cholesterol-rich egg yolks removed. You could order an egg white omelette in restaurants too. But as it turns out, there was absolutely no point at all in eating such things. A waste of your time. Indeed, you were missing out on all the good nutrition in the egg yolk.

Many researchers are now linking the development of heart disease to consistently high levels of an amino acid called homocysteine in the blood. This has been led by a dude called Kilmer S. McCully, which sounds like the kind of name someone who worked on *Rolling Stone* in 1968 would have had doesn't it? A colleague of Hunter S. Thompson, perhaps. 'Hey man, did you read McCully's piece on putting acid in Nixon's coffee?' Well, it does to me, anyway.

His work focuses on not just what you eat but the balance of nutrition as crucial to keeping the development of homocysteine low. He's very much against processed food, though is by no means a low carber. His theories outdate the cholesterol hypothesis which the statin industry services so profitably. How long before it is abandoned is anyone's guess, but as the money falls out of statins from 2012 when the patents expire, it may be sooner rather than later, especially if the drug companies can develop a drug that lowers homocysteine and repeat the massive profits they made on statins. It would be the pharmaceutical equivalent of how the music industry resold us our record collections on overpriced CDs, then on Mini-Discs and now as downloads. However, as it appears homocysteine can be kept low by a combination of diet and, if needed, simple vitamin supplements, this will take all their powers of marketing to achieve. They're probably working on it right now.

To say all this is confusing and a little disorientating is an understatement. But after a lot of consideration, I take a down-to-earth view. Let's face it, well before anyone had heard of cholesterol or saturated fat or pretty much anything else, people were often living well into their eighties. Up until the early twentieth century, if you made it to adulthood, you mostly died from bacterial infections or violent trauma i.e. some sort of pox or a tonne of pig iron falling on your head.

Lifestyle illnesses were not often a problem, especially for the working class; sometimes because the bacteria or violent trauma got to you first or more likely because such things were not prevalent among the bulk of people. Something has obviously changed in the mid and late twentieth century onwards and broad-brush advice such as eating less saturated fat – something humans have eaten for millennia – just does not make any sense. You'd think humans had not been able to survive at all before the invention of branded 'heart healthy' foods, that the human race was dying out until Flora margarine was invented.

Take a look around any Victorian graveyard and you'll see people who died in their seventies and eighties quite routinely. They must have lived off a diet wholly derived from animal fat – processed foods, vegetable oils etc. didn't exist commonly until well into the twentieth century and neither did margarine. Their introduction coincides with a big increase in coronary heart disease.

If saturated animal fat is such a threat to all our health, how come they lived so long? There was no dietary advice, no medicines, no nothing, but they still managed to live a long life. Indeed, there is a growing body of opinion that considers the very foods that replaced the 'old-fashioned' foods such as butter, lard and beef fat: that is to say, vegetable oils, polyunsaturated margarine and spreads are actually the real health problem. It is these unnatural foods that have caused the degenerative diseases that are now so common. The organisation at the forefront of this viewpoint is The Weston Price Foundation. They say that most cases of heart disease in the twentieth century are of a new form , namely a heart attack known as a myocardial infarction – a massive blood clot leading to obstruction of a coronary artery and consequent death to the heart muscle. They say myocardial infarction (MI) was almost non-existent in the United States in 1910 and caused no more than 3,000 deaths per year in 1930. Dr Paul Dudley White, who introduced the electrocardiograph (ECG) machine to the US, stated during a 1956 American Heart Association televised fundraiser: 'I began my practice as a cardiologist in 1921 and I never saw an MI patient until 1928.' However, by 1960, there were at least 500,000 MI deaths per year in the US. It surely can't just be a coincidence that this happened as the US embraced a new food culture based on increasingly large portions of highly processed foods, sugar and vegetable oils can it?

Vegetable oils have been the market leaders of fats for years and they've been pushed as 'heart healthy' because they're much higher in polyunsaturated and monounsaturated fats and lower in saturated fat. Many consider this to be actively dangerous and one of the core reasons behind so many degenerative diseases today. One of my favourite writers on this is a guy called Mark Sisson, author of *The Primal Blueprint*. He's one of these Californian guys who lives in Malibu, runs on the beach every day and generally lives the life of a surf-dude despite being fifty-seven. It's about as far away as possible from living in the suburbs of a British market town with 200 days of rain a year to live through. However, his research into these issues is very interesting. He says:

> PUFAs (polyunsatured fatty acids) can be a real Jekyll and Hyde. On the one hand, PUFAs include the essential fatty acids, including our favourite omega-3s. But when oxidation comes into play, we're looking at a whole different animal. Heating in particular sets a bad course in motion, but simple exposure to air, light and even moisture can incite the process. We're now looking at lipid peroxides, which initiate a free radical free-for-all. The free radicals make their way through the body pillaging at every turn. Their damage takes a toll on everything from cell membranes, to DNA/RNA strands, to blood vessels (which can then lead to plaque accumulation). The harm adds up over time in the organs and systems of the body and can cause significant impact, including premature aging and skin disease, liver damage, immune dysfunction, and even cancer.

When you think about it, the idea that somehow we've all suddenly become sick from basic foods such as milk, cream, butter or red meat or chicken skin because of its saturated fat or its cholesterol content, which is the implication behind the modern dietary advice, is just obviously very, very silly. The viewpoint of the likes of Weston Price and Sisson, among many others, that we need a return to 'old-fashioned' fats such as butter, lard and duck fat and, more broadly, to a diet free from processed food is backed up by a study of the Victorian diet from 1850 to 1900, published in the *Journal of the Royal Society For Medicine* called 'An unsuitable and degraded diet?'

Researchers Judith Rowbotham and Paul Clayton discovered that the previous fifty years had been ones of poverty and limited food availability for the lower orders but from 1850 to the turn of the century, food became more plentifully available, and cheaper. Consequently, the health of the working class improved markedly and has yet, 150 years later, to really improve. The mid-Victorian gene pool was not significantly different to our ours today, yet their incidence of degenerative disease was approximately 90 per cent less, they say.

Once the dangerous childhood years were passed, however, Victorian contemporary sources (including regional variables) reveal that life expectancy in the mid-Victorian period was not markedly different from what it is today. Once infant mortality is stripped out, life expectancy at age five was seventy-five for men and seventy-three for women. The lower figure for women reflects the danger of death in childbirth or from causes that were mainly unrelated to malnutrition. This compares favourably with present figures: life expectancy at birth, reflecting our improved standards of neo-natal care, currently averages 75.9 years for men and 81.3 years for women. Recent work has suggested that for today's working-class men and women (a group

more directly comparable to the mid-Victorian population) this is lower, at around seventy-two years for men and
seventy-six years for women.

Wow. This is amazing. Did they achieve this by not eating
red meat, eggs or butter? Did they achieve it through introduction of low-fat spreads, soya oil or skimmed milk? Of
course not. In fact they ate over 4,000 calories a day, fuelled
by lots of potatoes and bread, though not much sugar. They
had incredibly physically hard lives, working up to fourteen
hours a day in tough, labour-intensive work. The authors
discovered that their diets were rich in whole fish, especially
herring, featured lots of locally grown organic seasonal
vegetables and fruits. Organic not because they were all the
middle-class, collar-less shirt and homespun jumper types
called Jeremy and Clarissa who wanted to be 'like, totally
natural', but because chemical fertilisers and pesticides
hadn't been invented.

Meat on the bone, stewed or fried, was the most economi-
cal form of meat, generally eked out with offal meats including brains, heart, sweetbreads, liver, kidneys and 'pluck' (the
lungs and intestines of sheep). Pork was the most commonly
consumed meat. All meats were from free-range animals.

Milk was widely consumed but not usually in large quantities due to cost and adulteration fears. Butter consumption
was low due to the high cost for 'good' butter; lard and dripping were consumed routinely. Hard cheeses were favoured
by the working classes as a regular part of their diet. Their
long shelf life provided a stable protein source.

Rowbotham and Clayton found that this peak of good
health began to decline around 1900 with the introduction
of the first processed foods and when sugar became cheaper.

It is quite shocking to realise that, for most people,

longevity has not increased much since those times. No, not even skimmed milk and low-fat spread – which has been so common for the last twenty years – has made any difference. In fact things have, in real terms, got much worse.

We have a much higher incidence of heart disease than they did 150 years ago and we keep people alive with drugs and treatments not available to the Victorians. Despite the so-called healthy dietary advice for the last thirty years, the incidence has not dropped.

Gary Taubes makes a fascinating point about this in his seminal work *Good Calories, Bad Calories*:

According to the USDA, we have been eating less red meat, fewer eggs, and more poultry and fish; our average fat intake has dropped from 45 per cent of total calories to less than 35 per cent and National Institutes of Health surveys have documented a coincidental fall in our cholesterol levels. Between 1976 and 1996, there was a 40 per cent decline in hypertension in America, and a 28 per cent decline in the number of individuals with chronically high cholesterol levels. But the evidence does not suggest that these decreases have improved health. Heart disease death rates have indeed dropped over those years ... but there is little evidence that the incidence of heart disease has declined, as would be expected if eating less fat made a difference.

This was the conclusion, for instance, of a ten-year study of heart disease mortality published in *The New England Journal of Medicine* which suggested death rates are declining largely because doctors and emergency medical personnel are treating the disease more successfully.

He also goes on to say that as smoking rates have fallen from 33 to 25 per cent in this period this should have significantly reduced the incidence of heart disease and that therefore other lifestyle choices must have balanced it out. Given the widespread consumption today of such 'healthy' foods as low-fat spreads, given the decline in sales of butter and lard, given the widespread use of vegetable oils instead of animal fat for frying, surely, if these lifestyle choices were really efficacious, we'd have seen a change. But we haven't.

I find the report on the Victorian diet and life expectancy to be very pertinent because my grandparents were born at the end of that era. They were very against what they used to call 'fancy modern foods' and they'd say it in as strong, disparaging, sour Yorkshire tones as possible. There was nothing worse than fancy modern foods, except perhaps 'fancy foreign muck'.

They were born at the turn of the century into classic working class, labouring and very poor families in East Yorkshire and their food habits would have been inculcated in them by parents born in the 1870s, who in turn had been brought up by parents born in the 1840s.

This culture meant they simply considered anything that was made outside of the house to be inferior to anything they made themselves. Homemade was de facto best. They would not entertain processed food even though such processed food as there was hardly amounted to very much compared to today's bacchanalian feast of factory-made fodder.

They even ate very little canned food and when they did, in the case of corned beef, tinned ham or luncheon meat, all three of which are processed, it was still not considered the equal of fresh meat. It was used as a back up, often for Sunday tea when fresh wasn't available to be bought that day.

They had a strong food culture that was held as a moral code as well as a nutritional one. Sitting up straight and clearing your plate was seen as a duty. It put you closer to

God. To be a dilettante about your food was seen as morally weak and reprehensible. 'Don't just push your food around your plate, our John, it's not there to play with,' they'd say, disapprovingly.

Gran would talk disparagingly about people who she'd heard didn't have a big appetite or who were fussy eaters. 'He doesn't eat much,' was often said as though it showed a weak character or constitution.

But it didn't stop there.

My gran was vehemently against margarine and would only put butter on her bread. She would often say, 'I'm not eating anything made in a factory. You don't know what they put in it,' and among her own generation she wasn't alone in that fear. She would only fry in lard or beef dripping and considered the modern trend for cooking in oil as disgusting. Every meal came with great piles of vegetables, especially brassicas such as cauliflower, broccoli and cabbage. Cabbage was never far from any meal and if there was any left over it was used in bubble and squeak the next day. All vegetables were eaten only in season because that's only when they were available.

Every plate was loaded with potatoes and big hunks of bread were often used to mop up gravy. The bread was often home-baked, though she did buy Hovis a lot (I think she liked the adverts with the kid pushing a bike up a hill, which, if my memory serves me, was actually down south rather than some northern heartland as implied).

She would also make steamed sponge puddings served with lots of custard. It was a diet, like those of their parents, designed to keep people going through a long day's hard graft. Grandad Fred was a miner. You couldn't spend twelve hours underground in the West Yorkshire coalfield fuelled by salad and bean sprouts. Even in his sixties he was wiry and just incredibly strong. You wouldn't think it to look at him. He was quite short but he was all lean muscle and had a handshake strong enough to break a horse's leg, despite the fact he was missing two fingers on his right hand from an accident down the pit.

Just like the Victorians in Clayton and Rowbotham's study they had, by luck or good judgement, developed a diet that totally suited their lives. As a kid I thought this rigour and discipline towards food was simply part of their parochial, conservative outlook on life. It seemed to me they were stuck in a rut and wouldn't progress. They were living in the past. And that is all true. They were. Their culture was narrow and conservative, they didn't travel or have much experience of any other culture. This wasn't a self-made lifestyle choice. You got the life you got. Choices were few and far between. However, that didn't mean they knew nothing. They certainly knew what to eat to service their lives properly.

Their diet was high in carbs to fuel amazing amounts of physical work but it was also as diverse and varied as the seasons would allow. They were not picky or faddy eaters and they ate lots of cholesterol, saturated fat and animal fats. The portion size they ate was enough but not enough to make your belly hurt. It was modest because there wasn't money for excess food.

My gran lived until her late eighties(despite being a voracious smoker since a teenager) and Grandad Fred into his mid seventies despite a lung condition from breathing the coalfield dust for fifty, count them, fifty damn long years. That's what took the old bugger from us, not some lard induced heart attack. So clearly they thrived on this old-fashioned, saturated-fat diet. It was not unhealthy for them, so why should it be so now? Clearly, we don't need the rocket-fuel levels of carbs to give us fourteen hours worth of physical labouring energy but I can now see that everything else was a sensible and wholesome diet.

When I look back to my grandparents, they knew that all of these foods were actually what made them strong and healthy. This wasn't medical knowledge; it was born out of generations of lived lives. They knew not only what gave them health and strength but also what not eating these foods could do to you.

Their own grandparents lived through a period of starvation for the early Victorian working class and doubtless told tales of those days. They knew what they had lacked and how ill it had made people. Christ, if they could see people queueing up to buy skimmed milk today, they'd think everyone had lost their minds. Getting rid of the best bit of milk? Lunacy. I recall even late in her life Gran rejecting completely the advice on limiting consumption of eggs and looking in astonishment as Graham Kerr, the 'Galloping Gourmet', an early TV cook who was concerned about healthy eating, made an egg-white omelette. 'He's a bloody fool, that man,' she said, unequivocally, arms folded and a look of grim thunder on her face.

Obviously, a couple of anecdotes about long-lived relations do not an in depth scientific study make, but they were not unusual.

I'm hesitant to say granny knew best. It sounds crass and clichéd and I don't want to paint them as saintly or somehow faultless. As I said earlier they were pathologically anti-anything foreign or perceived as foreign. They were not adventurous in eating and had no food aspiration as we would know it. They had a very established, ingrained food culture which dictated food be wholesome and yet usually quite plain. Fancy it was not. Bloody hell no. And they were proud of it!

Yes they were culturally narrow but I'm now convinced that they knew something quite innately that we've forgotten or had brainwashed out of us by decades of bad health reporting, bad science, commercial interests and marketing. They knew what was good food and what wasn't.

Their generation suffered incredible hardship. They didn't live in a comfortable, centrally heated world. They were often cold and were almost always poor. They lived through two hellish world wars. Two! They couldn't afford health care of any sort until the establishment of the NHS in 1948, yet still, against the odds, they grew up lean and strong enough after all that to wield a pick all day long, three miles underground, hacking coal in unimaginably awful conditions.

And yet they didn't die of heart attacks. They didn't have food intolerances, they didn't have any of the modern degenerative diseases so common now. They were, frankly, tough bastards and did not suffer fools gladly. They would hate the twenty-first century faddy, paranoid and fearful attitudes to food. When I was about nine or ten I had, for no good reason, decided that I no longer liked beetroot. My mother had pandered to this whim but Gran would not have it. 'Get it eaten, it's good for you, it'll make you strong. It's a sin to leave food,' she would say and she'd stand over me until I ate it.

They did not tolerate fussy eating at all; in fact, they took rejection of any food offered as a personal insult. You really were not allowed to dislike a food: if they thought it was fresh and edible, you pretty much had to eat it and anyone who didn't or who had 'fancy ways' was frowned upon. They treated food as almost holy. On reflection I think this is because they knew quite viscerally that it was what gave them life and allowed them to live their life. They didn't take it for granted because starvation was in their folk memory. It mostly wasn't an indulgence or a treat, it was sustenance.

Do you think they would they have been stronger or lived longer lives if they'd eaten freakin' Benecol margarine to lower their cholesterol levels or fried in sunflower oil instead of lard?

We don't have to live such a tough life thankfully, but we can learn from their no-nonsense attitude to food and eat pure, unprocessed food cooked from scratch. It's our heritage in a way that low-fat spreads and bloody skimmed milk just are not.

Because of that, everything I have subsequently learned about diet and everything I eat myself has been put through the grandparent test. Partly out of fun but also to test it against their generation's food knowledge, a knowledge not influenced by TV ads or newspaper or magazine stories to the extent that ours is. What would they think of our diet?

They would have been scornful at us today with our food worries and paranoia. It was simple and clear to them. Meat and at least two vegetables at every meal. Lots of butter and full cream milk (they would have scorned yoghurt as little more than 'off' milk), bread, potatoes, cake and puddings. Nothing would have swayed them from that view, not even a doctor's advice. Had a low-fat diet been suggested by a doctor, Gran would have sneered at him and would have told him to his face that it was all rubbish, that you needed plenty of fat to 'keep the cold out'.

That seems less likely today. I'm sure most people think the official advice from their doctors about consumption of saturated fat is 100 per cent certain and foolproof. I know I did, but it's far from the truth. One day while writing this book I heard a Danish doctor on the radio talking about the country's new tax on saturated fat in food. He said, quite unequivocally that 'we know saturated fat is bad for us'.

Oh yeah? Think again, Jorgen. In Hannah Sutter's superb book *Big Fat Lies* she says France has a 0.2 per cent rate of death from coronary heart disease (CHD) – the lowest in Europe – and yet they have the highest consumption of saturated fats and the highest amount of people who do no exercise. The UK, often painted as the evil slob of Europe by those who love a bit of self-loathing, eats less saturated fat and does more exercise and yet has more CHD. The French also smoke more than us. If the advice on saturated fat were true, there'd be piles of dead Frenchies on every corner. There isn't. One speculated reason why there isn't, is because they eat more natural animal fats rather than vegetable oils and they cook meals from freshly bought ingredients rather than eat fast or processed food. In other words, they eat like we used to.

In Gascony, famous for its duck dishes and for the mass consumption of delicious duck fat (35 per cent saturated fat), the deaths from heart attacks are nearly half that of the rest of France and nearly 75 per cent less than the almost duck fat-free America. Try telling your doctor that you'll be giving up sunflower oil for duck fat and they'll punch you in the face – OK they won't, but they'd like to. It's madness. You'll die! Not if you're a Frenchman apparently. You've gotta love a duck.

I quit taking my statins eighteen months ago. Nothing bad has happened. Quite the reverse – I'm stronger and fitter and healthier. I am no longer at risk of all the other conditions that statins can cause or exacerbate. I don't want to be medicated for the rest of my life on the off chance that it might prevent a heart attack. I'd rather take my chances by living an active life and eating pure, natural foods. Does it seem crazy that I'd rather do that than mess with my body chemistry? Should I take powerful narcotics to try to remove something that my body actually needs in order to repair itself properly?

Although I'm sceptical about, in this case, the negative effects of saturated fat and cholesterol on our health when not hosed into us in industrial quantities, there are bound to be occasions and instances when, for specific individual reasons, they do affect people's health. In other words, while there are general principles which might apply to the majority, there are bound to be exceptions to any rule you want to draw up.

I think to really understand what works for our bodies we need to keep an open mind, even towards those ideas that we think the most objectionable. I say this having smugly thought I had healthy eating sorted by being a Mr Wholefood-Vegetarian. I'd closed my mind to any other point of view because it made life easier and didn't threaten my personal orthodoxy. Had I been more open-minded, I'd have got well sooner and I would never have eaten the bloody heinous creation that is soya cheese! And a life without soya cheese is, believe me, a better life.

IMITATION OF LIFE

'Soya bacon?'

'Soya bacon?!' she repeated louder and with more incredulity this time. It was as if I'd walked into Sainsbury's and asked for a pair of cheese trousers.

'Are you sure?'

'It does exist, honestly,' I said, somewhat affronted that my request was being voiced loudly for what seemed like the amusement of other Sainsbury's shoppers.

She looked at me with an expression 55 per cent 'Why is this long-haired grebo wasting my time?' and 45 per cent, 'Christ, it's a nutter who wants to stab me.'

This wasn't going well but I was committed to it now.

'What does it look like?'

'It looks a bit like bacon,' I said, helpfully adding, 'It comes in green packets.'

'Well the bacon section is over there.'

'Yes but it's not bacon, it's a vegetarian product made from soya. Do you stock it?'

'We just have *normal* bacon,' she replied with a bitter finality that suggested no more conversation was going to ensue. She seemed to have taken the request almost as an insult.

Well into the 1990s this was a typical experience when trying to get hold of such obscure soya-based foods in mainstream food retailers. Nowadays they'd not blink twice. 'Of course we have soya bacon, sir, it's a big seller among the health-conscious shopper and would you like to buy some soya capsules to lower your cholesterol while you're here as you look like a nice middle-class sort of chap?' Back then it was more a case of 'Oh shit, here comes the bloody hippies.'

As we've got more and more paranoid about cholesterol and animal fat, so the processed food industry has risen to the challenge of making money out of products that contain less or none of these evils. In the last twenty years the 'healthy' tag has been applied to everything and anything that is low in saturated fat and cholesterol.

Being able to make a health claim about your product is worth serious coin. Healthy options, or at least the options labelled healthy, are often more expensive. Healthy eating is an upmarket pursuit; it's aspirational and makes you look good. Look at yourself, filling your basket with healthy eating products, how brilliant are you? Not like the scum with the pizzas and the beer in their basket. You're looking after yourself, doing it right, one of the good guys. This is what the healthy eating foods shout to us from across the supermarket aisle.

All of that positivity doesn't come for free. You have to pay for it.

At the forefront of this new industry is the vegetarian option, especially the soya-based vegetarian option. Soya burgers, sausages, pies and the like. These days every supermarket does its own brand of these creations as well as stocking the alternatives. You will almost certainly eat some soya today in some form or other and it will be sold to you as being really healthy.

For years now, soya has been pushed as a healthy alternative to meat; it's being pushed as a healthy alternative to milk; it's being pushed as a healthy alternative to cheese; it's being pushed as a healthy alternative to cooking with lard; it's being pushed as a healthy alternative to breathing fresh air. You can get a soya version of everything these days. You can even probably get a soya version of sex. Sex without the meat.

Is soya protein, oil and milk really better than the traditional, well-produced animal versions? If I run it past my grandparent test I can tell you that it fails miserably. They would have said, 'What's wrong with proper food? That's just made-up rubbish that someone has invented to make money.' And they would be right. I've got a lot of soya history under my belt. If anyone knows anything about eating soya, it's me. I'm a bloody soya expert. I would wager that no one reading this, not one person, has eaten more soya foods than me. For twenty-six years I ate them several times every day without one day's break. Not one. Not in twenty-six years.

There isn't a soya-based foodstuff that I haven't eaten. Everything from tofu to tempeh, soya milk, soya ham, soya schnitzels, soya sausages, soya burgers, soya puddings, soya mince, soya steak, soya bacon, soya turkey, soya ham, soya beef, soya chicken, soya meat pies, soya pork pies, soya sausage rolls, soya cheese, soya ice cream, soya yoghurt, soya cream, soya margarine, soya duck (yes, really) and even soya bloody tuna. There isn't a soya product available in Britain that I have not eaten and eaten to excess. I think I loved them all, except the cheese which is an unholy creation, looking and smelling like something that would leak out of a dog's bottom.

Soya is massive. It is everywhere. According to the Institute of Food Research, soya is now a global staple food and about 220 million tonnes of beans are produced annually, mainly in the United States, Brazil and Argentina. European oil mills process about 16 million tonnes of soya beans annually, mostly imported from the US and Brazil. Soya beans and their products account for 27 per cent of US agricultural exports to the EU and were worth more than $2.5bn 2004.

Wow. That's a lot of soya but you might think this isn't much to do with you because you don't eat any soya products. You're not one of those veggie weirdos with dreadlocks and hemp trousers who eats those faux meats.

This may be true but, regardless, one way or another you almost certainly do eat soya because if you eat processed food of any kind it will almost always be present in some form or other, usually as soya flour but also as soya-protein concentrates, soya-protein isolate, hydrolyzed-vegetable protein, textured vegetable protein or soya lecithin. Mmm, delicious.

By processed, I simply mean food you didn't make yourself. Anything made in a factory rather than your own kitchen. This is the vast proportion of the stock of every supermarket in the western world. You'll find it in almost all commercially produced bread; it's in pastry, cakes, pies, confectionery and biscuits. You'll also find it in ice cream, most margarines and low-fat spreads as well as things like mayonnaise, salad cream, salad dressings and stock cubes.

And when it's not on duty as a foodstuff, it's working as an ingredient in paint, mattresses, industrial lubricants, carpets and inks. Well what foodstuff isn't? I've got a motorbike made out of carrots, me.

Henry Ford, who was a big soya nut, actually made a car out of soya-based plastic way back in 1941 when the rest of us were fighting the Nazis. Perhaps we should have used soya cheese as a secret weapon to kill the Hun. You couldn't eat the soya car, though. Well you could have but I imagine it would have been somewhat indigestible.

Once you become aware of it, you'll be amazed at just how frequently you're eating soya without realising it. Just check the labels on the stuff you regularly buy and you'll find it crops up everywhere. For example, if you go to the chip shop and if they say they use vegetable oil, it will almost certainly be soya oil.

Ah yes soya oil. It sounds so natural and healthy doesn't it? It should do, the soya industry has spent a fortune over the last fifty years trying to get that idea into our heads

Contrary to what you might think, you can't just squeeze a soya bean and get oil out of it. It takes a lot of work as it does for many other vegetable oils. For a couple of decades I bought the idea that soya oil was a simple, natural product. Just because I was told it was and I was told it was better for me than old-fashioned lard.

I certainly never realised a lot of oils are extracted in a complicated and elaborate industrial process using solvents. Do you really want to eat something that takes such effort to extract when simple, more natural alternatives are available; natural fats that have been eaten for millennia? Beef fat, lard, goose fat or butter are by comparison so natural and easily obtained. But we've been trained into thinking these are bad and that a highly contrived oil is somehow more natural and better for us.

This is how you get oil out of soya beans. It's about as far away from the stripped pine shelves of your local organic wholefood shop as you could imagine. I bet no one in the soya-oil factories has the dreadlocks and the hemp pants either.

The soya beans are cleaned, dried and dehulled prior to oil extraction. The soya bean hulls needs to be removed because they absorb oil and give a lower yield y'see. This de-hulling is done by cracking the soya beans and mechanically separating the hulls and cracked soya beans. Magnets are used to separate any iron from the soya beans. Yes magnets! This is already sounding more like a process to make kryptonite. The soya beans are heated to 75°C to coagulate the soy proteins and allow them to give up their oil more easily. It sounds like the beans are not overkeen on surrendering their oil.

First the soya beans are cut into flakes, which are then put into something called a percolation extractor. Then they are put into a solvent, usually hexane. Mmm, delicious hexane. Who doesn't love a snort of good old hex? After removing the hexane, the extracted flakes only contain about 1 per cent soya bean oil and it's this stuff which is used as livestock meal or transformed into the soy protein you find in your Linda McCartney-style products. The hexane is separated from the soya bean oil in evaporators. Are you keeping up? I'll be asking questions later.

Now they've got some soya oil but it needs cleaning up because it contains so many impurities. The oil-insoluble materials are removed through filtration and the soluble materials are removed by several different processes including degumming, alkali refining and bleaching, as any good wholesome food should, eh! Then they put it in a nice bottle, put a 'hey-this-is-so-natural' label on it and send it off to the hippies in the health food store and the nice middle-class shoppers in Waitrose. The job's a good 'un.

It shows you just how much money there must be in soya oil doesn't it? How cheap and plentiful it is for them to go to such an elaborate effort and then market it as a health food. Imagine how much energy is expended to get it from field to bottle. It seems like a lot of effort compared to say, olive oil. Crush an olive under the foot of a peasant and you're pretty much done. It's a world away from that and yet it's sold as though it's on the same 'natural' level as olive oil when, clearly, it just isn't.

Soya oil and other vegetable oils have been sold to us as 'heart healthy' because they are high in polyunsaturated fats. However, it is this very fact that many believe makes then very, very bad for us indeed.

In his book *The Inflammation Syndrome*, author Jack Challem says 'conventional cooking oils such as corn peanut, safflower soybean, sunflower and cottonseed oils are high in pro-inflammatory omega-6 fatty acids and contain virtually no anti-inflammatory omega-3 or omega-9 fatty acids'. As most of the fat we eat these days is vegetable oil, he argues this is causing widespread inflammation in the population, leading to all the degenerative diseases that are commonplace today. The typical western diet is radically out of balance between omega-3 and omega-6. We need omega-6 but we eat way too much. The ideal balance is said to be around 4:1 in favour of omega-6, but the typical western diet of starchy and processed foods is around 30:1 or higher. But it doesn't stop there, most commercially produced meat and fish is fed on wheat and soya. Both are rich in omega-6 and make the imbalance worse and worse.

Talking about the effect of high heat on the polyunsaturated oils, Californian Diana Schwarzbein M. D states, 'Damaged fat molecules become cellular debris, clogging cellular compartments and in turn damaging those cells. This contributes to the accelerated metabolic aging process.' And who wants their cellular compartments clogged?

Probably the best summation comes from our old beach dude, Mark Sisson, in *The Primal Blueprint*. Discussing oils such as canola, cottonseed, corn, safflower, sunflower and all similar vegetable oils which are heated to high temperatures for deep frying, he says:

Many of these oils are considered polyunsaturated fatty acids (PUFAs), which have a variety of serious health considerations. The concerns stem from PUFAs long-chain fatty acids, which are unstable, quickly go rancid and are easily oxidised into your body. Consequently PUFAs have a pro-inflammatory effect and disturb homeostasis in many other ways. The endocrine system is especially vulnerable to the effects of PUFAs' ingestion, leading to symptoms like a slowed metabolism, low energy levels and sluggish thyroid function. Heavy consumption of PUFAs in the modern diet is blamed as a leading contributor to obesity, diabetes, heart disease, cancer, immune problems, arthritis and other inflammatory conditions.

As I spent pretty much all my adult life consuming these vegetable oils and ended up fat, tired and as sick as a dog, I'm inclined, naturally enough, to agree. Since I've stopped eating these oils, slowly but surely most of the pain in my joints has gone and all my mid-afternoon exhaustion has evaporated. I just feel so much better. So much stronger. I can't believe this is a coincidence and that it would have happened anyway. It would not.

But it doesn't stop there with the soya. Most beef and dairy cattle as well as pigs are also fed on it too. It's also fed to poultry, to egg-laying hens and to fish on fish farms. What progress. We are feeding foodstuffs to animals that could not ever have possibly consumed them in nature. What chance does a salmon have to eat soya meal while it's swimming its way up stream? None, unless a vegetarian drops their burger into the river by accident.

Does feeding them like this make much sense? I can see it from the farmers' angle. It's high in protein and so makes them grow quickly and, in dairy cattle, it helps produce more milk. Wheat, used as animal feed, works in a similar way. All of this means more money, more quickly. But at what expense to the produce and to our health?

Mark Sisson says grass-fed organically reared meat has between two to six times more omega-3 than meat from animals raised on fortified grains and soya. This means inflammation is not promoted and the body works better, is stronger and more likely to be healthy. This was certainly my experience when changing from vegetable oils to animal fat. As it's organic it is also free of pesticides, antibiotics and other toxins. Others object to animals and fish fed on wheat and soya purely in terms of taste. Floppy-haired TV cook, Hugh Fearnley-Whittingstall brought the issue of farmed salmon to attention on his show, declaring he'd never eat a farmed salmon and saying how flabby and inferior they are to their wild relations. When I saw this shortly after my diet change and as a newbie to the world of eating fish, I went to a fishmonger and took a look. Hugh's expensive Eton education has not gone to waste. He was right. You can tell which is which just by looking at them.

Your farmed fishy fella is soft, pappy and marbled with fat. He's been on the fish sofa too long hoovering up fast food and not doing enough swimmy-swimmy. He's also probably a weirdly bright colour because they often put dye in the meal they feed the fish to make them look bright and attractive, some might say fluorescent. So they're as orange as a Geordie lass on a Friday night out in Bigg Market.

By contrast, your wild salmon is a much less fatty, more firm, meaty, muscular beast and has a far superior, more developed flavour. So far, in my experience the same thing is true of all intensively farmed meat and poultry compared to grass-fed, free-range, pasture-fed meat.

Now if this high wheat and soya-feed lifestyle makes fish

and animals flabby, it seems fairly likely it would do the same thing to us doesn't it? A critic might point out that humans are not fish (even I spotted that, though I've a met a few who might be some weird hybrid) and might thus react differently when fed on soya. Maybe this is true but I wouldn't say it if the evidence wasn't all around us.

We have the first soya-fed generation and they're, frankly, a lardy bunch. While, clearly, this isn't *all* down to soya, it must be playing a significant part simply because of its omnipresence in the food chain. Let's also not forget that I became what I believe is medically defined as a 'fat bastard' on a soya-based diet.

If you eat grass-fed meat next to wheat and soya-fed meat, you will notice a huge difference. One is rich and deep in flavour the other just isn't. I had an almost virginal palate when it came to meat and I could tell the difference right away.

This intensive feeding of animals with soya protein is a relatively recent development. Soya was primarily grown in the USA for use as industrial oil right up to the end of the Second World War. It was largely only after the war that it began to be used for animal feed because the soya producers had a lot of soya meal left over from the oil and wanted to make money out of it.

First it was used as animal feed and then they developed it into TVP (textured vegetable protein) and other foodstuffs. This began a fifty-year-long campaign to transform soya from an initial industrial by-product into a useful cheap food extender, then into an essential vegetarian protein and now, in the twenty-first century, into a hip, cool, health food for the middle classes to enjoy and maybe even feel smug about. Hey, it's even being pushed as a cure-all drug too. What a long strange soya trip it's been.

Growing up in the 1970s, soya would make appearances on futuristic programmes such as *Tomorrow's World* where it would be presented as the food of the future, capable, once processed, of mimicking all manner of other foodstuffs and thus providing cheap, high-protein meals. It is often said that it is a complete protein but many dispute this saying it lacks two amino acids: methionine and taurine.

More importantly, soya is high in something called phytic acid, which basically makes it hard to digest and thus causes what our American friends call gas, but which we call farts. Much money has been spent on taking the fart out of soya by selective breeding and genetic modification but I have to say, not quite enough money if my digestive system was any guide.

We've come a long way since 1984 when I first started eating this magic bean. Back then soya had not really permeated the popular, western consciousness. However, in the non-meat-eating culture, soya was already an almost holy foodstuff. Long before the mainstream got the soya message, we hippy-food-weirdos drank soya milk and ate TVP and its close relation HVP, hydrolyzed vegetable protein. There are few products quite as contrived as TVP and HVP. Nuclear waste is possibly more natural.

TVP and HVP are by-products of soya-bean oil manufacturing and are made from the flour that is left after all the oil has been removed from the soya-beans. The flour is cooked under pressure, textured by an extrusion process, shaped into small nuggets, strips or chunks, dried, and packaged for sale. Hungry yet?

It may also have flavourings, salt, monosodium glutamate or colouring added. Rubbery and distinctly beany, you have to work hard to make it tasty. It takes on other flavours in stews but somehow always maintains its slightly sweet beany-ness with a texture that is more old slipper than fillet steak.

But at least nothing died to make it though, eh, veggies? Well, actually, that's not true. A lot of animals almost certainly died in the clearing of the land to grow soya and in the harvesting of it, up to and including a few primates in the South American rainforest. This death might be a by-product of the industry but if you're precious about life, and as a veggie I used to think I was, then let's be honest, it's all death isn't it? Whatever the intent, it all ends up as a corpse be it beef cattle, a field mouse or a Howler monkey called Derek.

Clearly the processed soya foodstuffs owe more to food science than to nature. Looking back, it's weird that as avowedly naturalista hippies, the unnaturalness of TVP and other soya products just didn't matter to us, just as it doesn't seem to matter to the new generation of wholefood-eating shoppers; the fact that it was plant-based seemed to make it 'natural' per se, to the herbivore it was like having your own supply of 'vegetable meat', high in protein and low in fat. This, we thought, was a very good thing and we were told that high protein, low fat was a very healthy thing to eat and you will still be told this today. So we thought we were right and the meat eaters were wrong. Welcome to my world of bent logic. But I see the same kind of logic today. People think eating soya isn't just good for them, it's good for the planet.

Soya has a lot of fans now, more so than ever before. It has been eaten in China and the Far East for thousands of years and they thrived on it – or so we thought (though as it's a communist state and most people live in distant rural villages with little access to the outside world for generations, I'm not quite sure why we thought that). What we failed to appreciate was that they ate soya almost exclusively as tofu, which is little more than the curds of ground soya beans and water, or as tempeh, which is fermented beans. I liked tempeh, even though it looks like a growth you'd find in a disused toilet. This is a long way from eating the contrived, industrialised form of soya we've been hoovering up for thirty years and it is often held to be the case that these more ancient forms of soya foods are actually beneficial to health when eaten occasionally. It certainly sounds more likely.

The trouble is though, lots of people are allergic to soya. By the late 1980s and early 1990s, soya allergies were being identified so frequently that legislation was eventually brought in to enforce its listing on food labels. Some say that one in eight people is allergic to soya, which is very high but could actually still under-report the true level.

The symptoms of soya allergy are similar to milk allergy and they include rashes, diarrhoea, vomiting, stomach cramps and breathing difficulties. While you might have all of these symptoms after a night out in Middlesbrough, it could just be that you have an undiagnosed soya allergy rather than an intolerance to Teesside's local delicacies: parmos and Cameron's Strongarm beer.

The traditional view is that it's kids who suffer most from soya allergy but these sort of symptoms are the kind of thing that many people have as a background condition and if they're not too extreme would probably never be recognised as soya allergies, especially if you only consume soya as a constituent of products such as bread or biscuits.

People tolerate such symptoms as just part of life and certainly wouldn't go to the doctors to report it, and even if they did, it's doubtful that the doctor would think it was a soya problem right away. So it's quite possible there is a large but hidden amount of soy allergy and even more intolerance among the western world. But these kinds of symptoms markedly reduce your quality of life on a daily basis and simply prevent life being as much fun as it should be.

I especially used to love Linda McCartney sausages and would happily eat three or four at a time. Without fail, within an hour of eating them, I would develop a bloated gut which was so hard at the top of my belly that it felt as though it would burst. I half expected an alien to poke its head out. I used to call this 'shelfing' because it created a ledge I could virtually balance a pint on. While I got a similar response after many meals, it was always most profound after the sausages so I assumed it was something in them causing it, but rather than soya, I noticed they contained rusk, a wheat by-product, and assumed it was that. I was soya blind. Incidentally, I notice that some of the Linda McCartney boxes now have a picture of Paul in a flowing wheat field, arms outstretched. Surely, it would be more appropriate if he was in a limitless expanse of soya beans in an ex-rainforest in South America, arms outstretched as a family of monkeys look on, tears in their eyes.

We have no history of consuming so much synthesised, processed soya as we do today and so we have no idea what it might or might not do to us. How can we? We are effectively being experimented on by the processed-food industry, not against our will exactly, but probably to a greater extent than many realise.

As a vegan, I was a soya guinea pig for twenty-six years. This didn't involve running around a giant wheel much but it did involve eating soya every day. If it's going to mess with anyone, it'd be me and Dawn. And look what happened to us. The two conditions soya's critics accuse it of provoking most is digestive disruption with consequent malabsorption of nutrients and, secondly, hypothyroidism.

I suffered from the first, Dawn from the second.

I can't definitively prove that soya caused both of these conditions. However, changing our diet away from soya coincided with huge improvements in both conditions.

We always assumed it was safe to eat – surely it wouldn't be legal if it wasn't, that's how we thought about it – but given the constantly evolving nature of these soya products, the quantities they are eaten in and their label as a main source of protein, how do we really know what it's doing to us?

It's not like our parents or grandparents ate it for generations. We're the first ones to eat it in such huge amounts and so frequently. It is worth underlining this again: barely a day will go by without most people eating at least some form of soya.

We do have some idea what happens when an animal eats a lot of soya from the farming industry. It causes hypothyroidism which in turn causes them to put on a lot of weight quickly.

The soya industry knows soya has been linked to hypothyroidism and spends a good deal of time and energy allaying the public's fears about it, saying that it's really only a risk in those predisposed towards hypothyroidism and that the risk can be offset by the correct intake of iodine.

Phew, that's alright then.

Hang on. Who the feck knows if they're consuming enough iodine?

And even on the off chance that you knew you were, you'd still have no idea if you're actually absorbing all the iodine in your diet because soya inhibits how you absorb nutrition. The high amount of phytic acid inhibits absorption of minerals especially calcium, magnesium, manganese, molybdenum, copper, iron and zinc. This went on to cause me a huge imbalance between copper and zinc. My guts were wrecked, I passed semi-digested food every day for many years and you don't do that without there being consequences for your nutritional welfare.

While there's plenty of argument about soya and how good or bad it is for us in general, there isn't much disagreement over the fact that soya consumption is definitely bad for some people. But exactly how bad it is, for which people, in what quantity and from what sources are the variables in play.

You could spend most of the next year reading up on all the various reports and studies into soya consumption and you still wouldn't know whether the bloody stuff was going to damage your health in the long run. Unless you're allergic to it – which does seem to be increasingly likely – you won't drop to the floor, clutching your throat, screaming, 'Argh, the soya's gone done me in, Mama,' if you have some today. But I certainly believe soya was one of the core drivers of my IBS issues and was behind Dawn's subsequent thyroid and depression problems. And I know from reading other people's experiences in various forums that we're far from alone in having suffered this way.

A bit of tofu or tempeh now and then is probably OK, but as for the rest of it, well it's just processed food isn't it, so don't eat it. Then you don't have to worry. The one thing we can say for sure, no one ever died through lack of soya. Your body is not crying out for some soya cheese. It really isn't.

Soya is a multi-billion dollar industry in which huge multinational companies have a lot invested. They form a very powerful lobby group, but it is an increasingly controversial business being at the cutting edge of genetic modification in particular because great swathes of rainforest in Brazil and also in Argentina are being cleared to grow soya beans for the world animal-feed market.

Ninety per cent of all soya grown goes to the animal-feed business and you'll find veggies use this as a way to excuse their consumption of soya. 'It's not us who are causing the deforestation; it's the beastly meat industry.' And they are right in a way. But they are still almost certainly eating soya products grown in those areas. It might be only 10 per cent of the market, but it's still a market and it's a growing one. Does its minority status excuse it?

So remember, if you buy intensively reared animals you are buying into the destruction of the rainforests but also if you drink soya milk, eat soya burgers etc., you are supporting an industry that is intrinsically part of the industry of animal farming via animal feeds. Your vegan/veggie dollar is working hard for the products of the slaughter industry.

In the last thirty years, the thirty years in which the west has become fatter and more sick in so many ways, soya consumption has grown exponentially, to the point where around two thirds of all processed food in the US contains soya and it will not be much different here in the UK.

The people who would look with puzzled eyes at me and Dawn as we ate TVP in 1984, now often welcome it as super-cool and funky. 'Hey dude, it's like meat that's not, like, from an animal, so it's like, y'know, not exploiting any animals, that's cool, right?' No, not really. There's nothing natural about not eating animals. If anything is part of nature, it is killing things to eat them if you can. The hunter and the hunted is the story of all existence.

Soya producers are usually mandated to pay a levy of 0.5 to 1 per cent of their soya income to their soya industry organisational body for marketing and publicity purposes, so the industry is never short of cash to fund campaigns, scientific research or anything else that will help push their cause.

Now that I've stopped eating any soya products, the whole

thing strikes me as totally barmy and I can't understand why it took me so long to realise that I was relying on such contrived, synthetic foods for protein. When you sit and think about it, it is a very, very bizarre thing to do: to eat such manufactured junk.

After all, there's no shortage of basic foodstuffs with which to make meals even if you are a non-meat eater. It wasn't even as if I was a lazy cook. I enjoyed cooking and would take plenty of time to do it, but there was something almost compulsive about the fast food and it delivered a flavour and texture that I couldn't get anywhere else.

I'd speculate that this was in part due to the addition of what are usually labelled 'natural flavourings'.

You might wonder what a natural flavouring is. In this era of incredibly detailed labelling you might expect to read exactly what those natural flavourings are. Doesn't seem unreasonable, everything else is listed, why are the 'natural flavourings' exempt? Forgive me if I'm a bit cynical about it. Everyone who sells processed food is very keen to tell you their ingredients when they think it makes them look good, so conversely, the only reason not to tell us what the natural flavourings being used are is presumably because they fear it will make them look bad.

It also allows them to protect their brand so competitors won't know what makes the product taste as it does. After all, processed food such as soya burgers have no flavour at all. Unlike meat, they need flavour added to them to make them edible. If the natural flavours in natural flavouring looked natural to us, they'd list them. The fact is it's probably a food laboratory creation with little more than a code name to identify it. And that doesn't look so nice on your wholesome green box of natural goodness. Hey man, I love these new IPSX4343265 flavour veggie sausages, so much nicer than the old DFDGG554565 variety.

In the US a natural flavouring is legally defined by the Code of Federal Regulations as:

> the essential oil, oleoresin, essence or extractive, protein hydrolysate, distillate, or any product of roasting, heating or enzymolysis, which contains the flavoring constituents derived from a spice, fruit or fruit juice, vegetable or vegetable juice, edible yeast, herb, bark, bud, root, leaf or similar plant material, meat, seafood, poultry, eggs, dairy products, or fermentation products thereof, whose significant function in food is flavoring rather than nutritional.

Imagine how many lawyers got rich drawing that up. All so that flavourings can be added to processed food. Mad.

For all of the packaging and warm words about how healthy they are, these soya foods are the most contrived, synthesised foods you will find anywhere. It's one thing to just say 'Sod it, I'll eat what I like' and gorge yourself on every breadcrumbed, deep-fried amalgam you want, but it's another to still think you're being healthy in doing so. And that's where I went wrong. I still thought this was healthy eating and the literature and government advice increasingly backed me up on this just as it still does today. While that literature will warn you about your fat, sugar and salt intake, there is never a word to say about anything that is added to processed food, be it flavourings, preservatives or artificial sweeteners.

Soya products are usually lower in saturated fat than their meaty alternatives; they are high in polyunsatured fats and lower in calories. They don't contain cholesterol either, as they will be quick to tell you on their packaging. Whoo hoo, yeah baby, that ticks all those paranoid food boxes your doctor wants ticked but we already know the whole cholesterol-in-your-food business is irrelevant.

There is so much money in soya and so many vested interests with profits to protect and money available to spend on lobbying to keep governments pushing the 'soya is healthy' advice, that any challenge to soya's supremacy will take a concerted effort or some overwhelming evidence that it makes you grow two heads, and even if it did, the soya industry would resell the two-heads side effect as a doubling of your mental capacity.

Across the last thirty years, the public have eventually been persuaded that soya is cool, hip and healthy and it may take another thirty to persuade them that in its highly synthesised forms it simply is not; rather it is potentially very destructive to good health. I should bloody well know. The thing is, I'm ahead of the wave on this, I know what soya can do to you long term. I've been out there to the edge of soya oblivion so you don't have to.

HE THOUGHT HE WAS A MAN
BUT HE WAS A MUFFIN

We were taking a month-long break in California in 2004 and were in the bar of the very lovely Portola Hotel in Monterey. A couple came in and took a couple of seats. It was table service, which I love – there's nothing more luxurious in life than having drink brought to your table. It's so much more sophisticated than having to queue at a bar like a beast waiting to be watered.

The waitress scoots over to take the couple's order.

'Do you have any low-carb beer?' he asks.

I turned to look at Dawn, who was drinking a tequila sunrise from a glass the size of her head. 'Low-carb beer?' I said, 'What the hell is a low-carb beer?'

'Sure, two low-carb beers coming up,' said the waitress in that happy to serve, positive tone that Americans so often provide with even the most basic service, bless them.

They had low-carb beer. Low. Carb. Beer. Those crazy Californians.

Around that time in 2004, low carb was everywhere in California. It was the hippest diet on the block and no menu was complete without several low-carb options, even in Denny's. People were obsessed with it and especially with the

Atkins Diet, now largely discredited. It seemed to come from nowhere, a magical new approach to eating which would make you lose weight without depriving yourself of much food at all; indeed, you could eat as much bacon, eggs and cream as you wanted. Hurrah, thought fat America, a chance to still overeat and yet lose weight. Hmm. That doesn't seem quite right, bubba. No, no it's true I tells ya!

No advert on TV was complete without a reassuring statement that whatever it was, was low in carbs, even if it was an ad for a Ford car, wrinkle-free Dockers or coal.

In the supermarkets everything had a 'low carb' statement on it, even things which had no carbs at all in them like fizzy water! Yeah low-carb fizzy water, as opposed to that starchy, high-carb water you normally get.

In our typically cynical, English way, we saw all this and said, what a load of old bollocks. It was so obviously a fad; a food fashion. It was so big, so omnipresent, it had nowhere to go but down.

By the time of our next California visit a year later, there was not a mention of low carbs on TV ads for foods nor was it mentioned on menus. It was as if it had never happened; like it was a love affair which, in retrospect, all parties were ashamed of and now chose to keep quiet about.

It was so last year, so last year in fact that the Atkins company had gone bust. It seemed that just as quickly as everyone had jumped on the bandwagon, they had jumped off.

It was the same over here in the UK, of course. Previously very fat people turned up on TV looking thinner and declared they'd done it by eating bacon and eggs and steak. Everyone was amazed, what weird magic was this?

It wasn't long before doctors and other health officials started warning about diets high in fat and low in carbs. All that saturated fat will increase your chances of a heart attack, blah blah blah, all the usual stuff, even though, in retrospect, there was little hard and fast evidence that this would be the case because there had been little in the way of research into the long term impact of low-carb, higher-fat diets. At the time they were still trying to pass off cholesterol consumption as Officially a Bad Thing That Could Kill You, even though, as we have seen, they have since backtracked on this advice. However, there were plenty of horror stories about people who went mental on this diet and ate a pound of bacon a day and washed it down with a pint of cream, presumably on the old Todd Rundgren principle that 'if a thing is worth doing, it's worth over-doing'.

There was also confusion over various no-carb, low-carb and lower-carb diets, which often ended up conflated under the low carb banner as though they were the same thing, with all subsequent health advice based on that confusion.

The industries that had most to lose by the widespread adoption of the low-carb lifestyle, primarily wheat and sugar-based food producers, had got to work on producing science to prove low-carb diets were bad, honestly they really are and not just because we're not selling so many donuts anymore. There was a brief but big panic as sales of pasta and rice in America dropped by over 8 per cent in 2004, which is a lot of dollars not falling into the bread basket. They need not have worried. The public were far more addicted to cheap carbohydrates than they had briefly thought.

People began to fall off the low carb wagon, presumably unable to find the discipline to permanently live a life without chips, bread and bowls of pasta. Consequently they often put all their weight back on again when they reverted back to the traditional diet, the same diet that had made them fat. Not sensible. But perhaps inevitable.

Even poor old Doc Atkins himself passed away. The urban myth is that he died of a heart attack. Of course, like Hitler being a vegetarian, this was just made-up nonsense. The old boy had fallen over and hit his head, in fact.

People stopped thinking low carb was a good way to lose weight and, more typically, got the idea that it was actually rather bad for you, which if you abused it, it certainly was. The official healthy eating advice was still pushing carbs as the thing to base your meals on, so everyone went back to the default setting and the panic was over, Atkins became FAtkins and was buried, just another corpse in the graveyard of fad diets. The pro-carbohydrate, low-fat orthodoxy was reasserted and still rules today and yes, people are still fat and getting fatter.

In recent years, it has re-emerged, zombie-like, and now sells all sorts of products many feel are a serious departure from the original ideas in Dr Atkins's first book in 1972. Today the resurrected brand sells snackbars, protein-shake powders and wholegrain bread mixes, and other processed, manufactured foods. It's pretty much indistinguishable from any other diet company selling made-up food.

Interestingly though, the low-carb lifestyle has moved on from the crazy days of fad diets, away from processed foods altogether, and has been reborn in a variety of strains as a more natural, wholesome diet based on real food. The fashion was over but eating less starch as an idea never really went away, rather it evolved. And it never went away because for a good many people it works. It works not just as a way to lose weight; it works as a healthy lifestyle. Sorry doctors, sorry NHS Eat Well plate, it doesn't matter what you say, or how you argue otherwise, it quite simply does and for thousands of people.

Many find a low-carb life is a life that gives you more

energy, more mood and emotional stability, more physical strength and more happiness. All the changes I experienced are shared and mirrored by many others. Today the low carb philosophy is deeper and wider than when at its trendy peak, so much so that some even call it a movement. Of course, many give it a go but still can't stick with it as a way of life and lapse back into the starchy diet. Inevitably it's not appropriate for everyone's body or lifestyle. I have to say, it works damn well for me.

Most of the surface area of your local supermarket is dedicated to pushing carbohydrate foods. Look at how much space the bread, biscuits, crackers, cakes, pasta, rice, sugar, breakfast cereal, pasties, and confectionery products take up.

Everyday and ordinary it might be, but this addiction to carbs is what a great many people consider to be behind the problems with our weight and health. However, while the alternative-eating army might well be largely united in their opposition to the mass consumption of carbs, this is far from the official healthy eating advice.

That NHS Eat Well website recommends you base your diet around starchy foods. They say:

> Starchy foods such as bread, cereals, potatoes, pasta, maize and cornbread are an important part of a healthy diet. They are a good source of energy and the main source of a range of nutrients in our diet. Starchy foods are fuel for your body. Starchy foods should make up around one third of everything we eat. This means we should base our meals on these foods.

This has pretty much been the advice for nearly the last thirty years. The thirty years in which obesity has risen dramatically. Well done NHS. Well done doctors. Keep your head down and pretend it's not happening. The fact is this advice either causes people to put on weight or it makes overeating so easy that it happens anyway.

But it's been drummed into us so much for so long by so many official medical sources that to question it and to go against it feels like a terrible heresy. As you know, I was Mr Wholegrains for years. I thought this put me on the side of the healthy-food angels. I based every meal I ate for thirty years on wholegrains and starches. Was that wrong? Yes it damn well was for me and I know it has been for many other people too. It won't suit everyone, but should we destroy the health of everyone else because of that?

It is incontestable that my health improved massively as soon as I changed my diet. I don't eat starchy foods like potatoes. I do occasionally, if I'm feeling freakin' crazy and adventurous, eat an oatcake or a spoonful of wild rice. That's as starchy as I get. And I have to tell you I have never been more healthy. I don't lack for nutrition because everything I eat is, unlike grains, nutrient dense. And I don't lack for fibre because I eat lots of vegetable matter. Other than to fill the belly, I can't see what I would get from grain that I don't get from everything else that I eat.

I'm not alone in this. Thousands of people have discovered that cutting out starchy foods and limiting carbs in general improves every aspect of their health. Why does the medical establishment and the government treat us all as if we have the same body that requires the same nutrition at the same time from the same sources? It makes no sense at all.

The NHS Eat Well plate, the one that says you should have 33 per cent of that plate piled up with starch, doesn't seem to realise or think it worth noting that as well as grains, all beans and pulses are also starchy carbohydrates. Not quite as starchy as a potato perhaps but full of carbohydrate nonetheless. They class these as proteins, which they are as well, of course, but if you eat, as I did for years, a lentil curry with rice, that is virtually an all-carb meal with very little protein, and what protein it does have is not high-class protein. This means all the things in your body that need the ten amino acids to work properly don't get them all and so don't.

They go on to say another third of your plate should be fruit and vegetables. Yeah, yeah, OK, does this mean for every meal? Can I have a whole plate some days? Can I skip a day? Will I die if I do? Hello? Hello? Is anybody in there? Just nod if you can hear me.

This is a strange generalisation anyway. All fruit and vegetables are not the same in terms of nutrition or in how you digest them; in fact they are all very different. Some are high in sugar and thus high in carbs too. For example, thirty grapes have about the same amount of carbs as a cup of potato whereas celery has almost no carbs. Just generalising the advice as though all fruit and vegetables will work the same way inside you makes no sense at all.

The Eat Well plate goes on to recommend that around 10 per cent of your diet should be sugars and fat with the rest being protein and dairy. But sugar works like a carb when it reaches in your digestive system. Dairy produce also contains some carbs. Oh and so do nuts and seeds too. They're not really high, like a potato; nonetheless, they're in there.

Roll all these things together and it's not hard to see this plate is a carbohydrate time bomb. By the time you've had your recommended 33 per cent of starch, some sugary fruits and veg, a glass of milk, some nuts and a sweet pudding of some sort, all you're really doing is taking in carbohydrate on a huge scale.

OK but who cares? What does it matter?

Far from being a modern bourgeois obsession, the benefits of not eating much carbohydrate have been known about for 150 years and of course our hunter-gatherer ancestors existed for thousands and thousands of years as low-carb eaters because there were only two branches of Nandos open at the time.

In fact until the early 1980s, it was common knowledge that if you wanted to lose weight, you should cut out potatoes, bread and rice. This was the advice, if you recall, to my dad from his doctor at the time. Proof that doctors don't always get it wrong! Today, the advice would be different. So, while many of the diets you'll find pushed by people are variations of low-carb eating, all that many are really doing is echoing previous understandings.

When I asked my friends who had lost weight how they or their friends had done it, all of them said via a low-carbohydrate regime, even if it was just cutting down on bread and potatoes. It still works. Fat doesn't make you fat, carbs do. While there are many, many alternative healthy eating ideas and diets, the one thing just about all of them are agreed on is that the Eat Well plate is just bad advice and that over-consumption of carbohydrate is causing obesity and the whole host of the degenerative diseases we see around us, especially combined with the inflammation provoked by the imbalance between omega-3 and omega-6 in the modern-day diet. Some even consider carbs help promote cancers and poor eyesight.

One of the odd physical consequences of the change in my diet was to radically improve my eyesight. For five years I had needed glasses for reading. About a month into my new diet I suddenly noticed that words that had been blurred were now back in focus. So much so that I stopped using glasses at all and I haven't put them on for nearly a year and a half now. My eyesight is not 20/20 perfect, the twenty-six healthy high-carb years years saw to that, but it's so much better than it used to be and I feel that it is slowly getting better still. This doesn't just happen does it? It can't be a weird coincidence; it must be diet-related – either that or I have been blessed by some kind of miracle. Which seems unlikely given my life of sin.

While researching this topic, I found there are a great number of people who have reported this phenomenon. It has been especially noted in the diabetes community when carbs are cut, some people even reporting 20/20 vision after years of wearing glasses. I assumed that bad eyesight was endemic to all human populations, just being some sort of 'natural' deterioration, but this may not be correct. Decline may be very much diet-related.

Barry Groves, who has researched such topics for many years talked about research into native tribes in his book *Trick or Treat*:

> In 2002 a group of scientists led by Professor Loren Cordain, an evolutionary biologist at Colorado State University, published a review of the literature. They looked at 229 hunter-gatherer tribes and confirmed that primitive populations had low rates of myopia even in those receiving formal education. It was all down to food. Cordain was clear that cereals were to blame. 'In the islands of Vanuatu', he said, 'they have eight hours of compulsory schooling a day. Yet the rate of myopia in these children is only 2 per cent.' The difference between them and Europeans was that the Vanuatuans ate fish, yam and coconut rather than white bread and cereals.

Experts interviewed by the BBC had mixed reactions to this review. Dr Nick Astbury, vice-president of the Royal College of Ophthalmologists, told BBC News Online, 'It's an interesting theory, but it needs more evidence to support it.' Although he did admit that the reasons for short-sightedness were 'multi-factorial', so diets high in refined starches could play a part. Furthermore, James Mertz, a biochemist at the New England College of Optometry in Boston, remarked, 'It's a very surprising idea.'

However, Bill Stell of the University of Calgary in Canada said, 'It wouldn't surprise me at all. Those of us who work with local growth factors within the eye would have no problem with that – in fact we would expect it.'

It would appear that when hunter-gatherer societies changed their primitive existence to a more western lifestyle and altered the type of food they ate, their eyesight began to deteriorate.

Well there's no question that my eyesight has radically improved.

However, it is obesity that concerns everyone more than any other issue. Given that I was fourteen and a half stone on my carb-based diet, and was heading towards fifteen with ease, I wanted to know how and why this happened. In carrying out my research I discovered more about the workings of my pancreas than any man whose real passion in life is rock 'n' roll and not medicine really should have to know.

The biology is all freely available if you want to look it up, however, this is a basic summation of how it all works from an actual real life doctor called Andreas Eenfeldt. He's a Swedish medical doctor specialising in family medicine, whatever 'family' medicine actually is. Concentrate, here comes the science:

All digestible carbohydrates are broken down to simple sugars in the intestines. The sugar is absorbed into the blood, raising the blood glucose. This increases the production of the hormone insulin. And insulin is our fat-storing hormone. Insulin is produced in the pancreas. In large amounts insulin prevents fat burning and stores surplus nutrients in the fat cells. After some time (a few hours or less) this may result in a shortage of nutrients in the blood, creating feelings of hunger and cravings for something sweet. Usually at that point people eat some more. That starts the process again, a vicious cycle leading to weight gain. A low intake of carbohydrates gives you a lower and more stable blood glucose, and lower amounts of insulin. This increases the release of fat from your fat stores and increases the fat burning. This usually gives fat loss, especially around the tummy in abdominally obese individuals.

This explains perfectly how and why I become fat. It is exactly what happened to me.

If starch is our primary fuel, we surely only need to take it in when we're going to be very active.

The amount of carbs you eat in a recommended diet is around 300g a day, though almost no one would ever be able to guess how much they'd eaten without weighing everything and looking up the carb content. The amount recommended on most alternative low-carb diets is 100g or less. I eat between fifty and seventy-five most days. If I've got a really physical day digging the garden or mowing our three-quarters of an acre of grass, sometimes I'll up it to around 100. This gives me all the energy I need, I don't get sleepy during the afternoons and I don't put on body fat despite the fact that I eat small amounts of thick full cream, butter and coconut oil every day.

Are we really to believe that a bloke who is five foot three tall and sits behind a desk all day should eat the same amount of carbs as a six foot two inch road digger? There is no allowance in the advice for such differences in body and lifestyle. Madness.

But it's not just the weight issue that improves by limiting your carbs. Possibly the best thing about it in my experience is climbing off the roller coaster of blood sugar peaks and troughs. It's fantastic to be free of the manic, over-emotional highs and the dozy, foggy-headed lows.

It has kept me even-tempered and headache-free now for eighteen months. Not one headache. This from a bloke who suffered from them almost daily until the day I stopped eating my healthy-vegetarian diet. How fantastic is that? What would you give to be headache-free?

However, I'm very aware that this way of eating is seen as weird and extreme not least because it means I don't eat bread or any wheat. Not eating bread. How wacked-out is that? Bread is so literally ingrained into our lives and our lifestyle that to live entirely without it seems deeply unnatural and extreme.

When I tell people I don't eat bread they assume it's because I'm gluten intolerant. Funny how everyone has heard of gluten intolerance these days isn't it? It'd be tempting to think that being gluten intolerant is almost fashionable.

Thirty years ago no one had heard of such a concept because as far as we knew no one seemed to be gluten intolerant. Someone must have been I guess, but it was not the common thing it is today, even allowing for misdiagnosis. Some estimates say just a decade ago gluten-intolerance levels were at one in 2,500 people worldwide. Today, it's at one person in 133. Something has changed hugely in a short space of time, though I'd have thought 1 in 2,500 was actually quite a high amount, let alone one in 133.

Until recently, gluten-free products were certainly not

found in supermarkets but now it's a big and growing business. Suddenly, everyone is intolerant of gluten – they just won't stand for gluten! But of course, I'm not gluten intolerant – or at least the tests I had at the doctors proved I wasn't. They could be wrong of course; it wouldn't surprise me if they were.

When I say I don't eat bread and I'm not gluten intolerant, a look of bewilderment crosses people's faces. Why would you not eat bread if you could?

'I couldn't live without toast,' one told me. 'My life would be much worse if I couldn't eat a bacon sarnie,' said someone else.

Yes, our lives have been set up to eat bread. When you walk into a supermarket you are confronted with a massive aisle of bread varieties. It'd be amazing if not eating bread didn't seem a very odd thing to do indeed.

But actually, once you decide not to, it is remarkably easy. Most bread that you eat most days isn't actually that fantastic anyway. It's often an almost tasteless wrapper for other stuff that provides very little satisfaction in and of itself

I've actually eaten bread three times since my change of diet just to see what it would be like. I've done the same thing with potatoes as well. After both I had bad, throat-burning indigestion. That, along with that 'full' feeling which isn't very pleasurable, was the main consequence.

The odd thing is, having spent so much of my life eating bread and potatoes, I thought eating them again would reawaken a passion for them and make me feel I was really missing out on some good stuff by not eating them. But the absolute reverse was true. They seemed largely flavourless, dull and now irrelevant.

So many of our eating habits are just that: habits. They're not choices really, they're just things we eat by default because we can't think of anything else. But life doesn't fall apart when you reject these common, everyday foods and when you feel so good in body and mind by doing so it is more than enough reward for making the effort.

However, as ever, I like to run this past my grandparents' generation to see what they would have made of it and I know fine well that they would have thought it a lunatic idea. 'Live without bread? 'Ave you gone soft in the 'ead our John? It's the stuff of life. It's in the Bible and everything. Bread doesn't make you ill, take a good hard look at yourself, lad.' That would have been the verdict. And for their lives – tough, physical lives – they'd have been right.

Of course, their generation and those that preceded them managed to eat a lot of wheat without suffering from the gluten intolerances and degenerative diseases we suffer today, and also without putting on so much weight. How come? Was it all down to them being much more active? This issue is addressed in a new book called *Wheat Belly* by Dr William Davis, who argues that it is the nature of the variety of modern-day wheat which is destroying our health, increasing intolerances and responsible for making us fat. He explains how modern wheat is a perversion of what wheat used to be:

> If you held up a conventional wheat plant from fifty years ago against a modern, high-yield dwarf wheat plant, you would see that today's plant is about two-and-a-half feet shorter. It's stockier, so it can support a much heavier seed-bed, and it grows much faster. The great irony here is that the term 'genetic modification' refers to the actual insertion or deletion of a gene, and that's not what's happened with wheat. Instead, the plant has been hybridised and crossbred to make it resistant to drought and fungi, and to vastly increase yield per acre. Agricultural geneticists have shown that wheat proteins undergo structural change with

hybridisation, and that the hybrid contains proteins that are found in neither parent plant. Now, it shouldn't be the case that every single new agricultural hybrid has to be checked and tested, that would be absurd. But we've created thousands of what I call Frankengrains over the past fifty years, using pretty extreme techniques, and their safety for human consumption has never been tested or even questioned.

He goes on to test old strains of wheat against new and discovers that the new raise blood sugar incredibly high and very quickly:

It [wheat] contains amylopectin A, which is more efficiently converted to blood sugar than just about any other carbohydrate, including table sugar. In fact, two slices of whole-wheat bread increase blood sugar to a higher level than a candy bar does. And then, after about two hours, your blood sugar plunges and you get shaky, your brain feels foggy, you're hungry. So let's say you have an English muffin for breakfast. Two hours later you're starving, so you have a handful of crackers, and then some potato chips, and your blood sugar rises again. That cycle of highs and lows just keeps going throughout the day, so you're constantly feeling hungry and constantly eating. Dieticians have responded to this by advising that we graze throughout the day, which is just nonsense. If you eliminate wheat from your diet, you're no longer hungry between meals because you've stopped that cycle. You've cut out the appetite stimulant, and consequently you lose weight very quickly. I've seen this with thousands of patients.

Oddly enough, just as I was reading his book, I found an old picture of me walking through a field of wheat in Oxfordshire in 1981. We were at the Cropredy festival to see Fairport Convention and had gone for a long walk. The wheat is shoulder high. Yet the wheat grown locally to me here in Norfolk is knee-high. The waving fields of wheat are much less, well, wavy than they used to be because these short straw varieties are now the norm.

If Dr Davis is right, it goes to the very heart of one of the biggest and most powerful businesses on earth. You can imagine the wheat lobby will have its scientists and well-funded ad campaigns wheeled out if it sniffs so much as a whiff of danger to its profits, just as they did in 2004 when, en masse, people stopped eating pasta and bread.

We feel instinctively that wheat is natural and wholesome but considering twenty-first century wheat is a modern creation, very different from its ancestors, the idea that it's some ancient, traditional food is turned on its head. Everyone in the industry pretends like it hasn't changed in the 5,000 years we've been eating it, like your daily loaf is little different from that baked by your ancestors in the Middle Ages, but nothing could be further from the truth. It's just another way that we've been led away from questioning the foodstuffs that are so commonplace and so omnipresent in our lives.

And of course, your wheat consumption doesn't stop at bread. In the same way soya is ever-present in modern processed food, so is wheat – in one form or another. You probably eat wheat at every meal and don't even think about it. A wheat-based cereal for breakfast, a sandwich for lunch, pasta for your evening meal and maybe some toast or cereal for supper. That's not including other snacks such as biscuits, muffins, crackers or anything with pastry. Pretty soon, when you eat like that, you become the Pillsbury Dough Boy; a muffin man of gargantuan proportions. Carbs are so easy not just to eat but to overeat. Even if we accept –

and I don't – that 300g was the right amount for you to eat, it's so effortless to eat a lot more than that, not least because it takes twenty to thirty minutes of eating carbs before you feel full – you can cram a lot of energy dense food into you in that space of time.

Dr Davis describes wheat as 'addictive':

National Institutes of Health researchers showed that gluten-derived polypeptides can cross into the brain and bind to the brain's opiate receptors. So you get this mild euphoria after eating a product made with wholewheat.

I have to say when I stopped eating wheat I didn't experience any kind of withdrawal symptoms at all. It was very easy to do, the only difficulty was that I was so habitual in my wheat consumption that for a few days, I didn't know what to eat at certain times of the day. No crackers or toast to rely on, it seemed odd. But quickly you get into new habits and break the old ones. Not having your usual default options for food does initially make you feel somewhat adrift in life but I found it very refreshing. I enjoyed the challenge of creating new food regimes and habits. It might seem difficult at first but it really isn't.

Since I stopped eating not just wheat but all other grains too, along with other high-carbohydrate foods such as potatoes and beer, I've felt liberated by the experience. I would recommend everyone try it for at least a week just to see how different it makes you feel.

The Eat Well plate will not entertain any of this rebellious nonsense; it's quite catty about low-carb diets, calling them 'a fad'. What a contrast to the Swedish government. On 16 January, 2008, the National Board of Health and Welfare declared that a low-carb diet is 'in accordance with science and a well-tried experience for reducing obesity and Type 2 diabetes'.

This is what Nanny NHS says:

> Some diets are very low in carbohydrates (such as pasta, bread and rice), which are an essential source of energy. While you may lose weight on these types of diets, they're often high in protein and fat, which can make you ill. It has been suggested that the high-protein content of these diets 'dampens' the appetite and feelings of hunger. Many low-carbohydrate diets allow you to eat foods that are high in saturated fat, such as butter, cheese and meat. Too much saturated fat can raise your cholesterol and increase your risk of heart disease and stroke.

They don't say why 300g is the correct level intake. They don't quote their sources or their science. Sorry, not good enough. How come I've got more energy eating around 70–100g of carbs a day? By this calculation I should have had more energy when I ate 400g per day. But the reverse was true. It all seems too poorly justified and simply false. To be honest, I think it's just made up by a committee. It's based on nothing more than supposition, guesswork and the need to say something, anything.

And they are wrong; it is rarely said by anyone in the low carb movement that protein suppresses appetite. It is almost always said, and it is 100 per cent true, that fat suppresses your appetite because it takes much longer to digest. This is documented time and again by people who have adopted the regime and it was almost the first thing I noticed when I changed my diet. For example, my breakfast today of smoked wild salmon, organic cream cheese, organic free-range poached eggs and organic wild rice followed by home-grown raspberries and organic double cream was low carb and quite high fat. I ate it at 8.30am and at 1.00pm I still wasn't hungry. My old carby breakfasts based on toast or cereal used to leave me hungry before midday. There is no acknowledgement of this at all by the NHS, possibly because it might make this high-fat diet sound too attractive.

We dealt with the wacky 'too much saturated fat can raise your cholesterol and increase your risk of heart disease and stroke' business in a previous chapter. This is all you've got against lower carb eating, is it NHS? It's hardly a persuasive, comprehensive or even well-researched argument is it? I'm not saying it's perfect for everyone but to dismiss it like this is astonishingly stupid. Why not, even for a moment, consider its popularity might actually have some core of truth or veracity about it? Why not entertain that as a possibility? After all, what have we got to lose? The current advice has failed. The next generation might live shorter lives than ours due to obesity and other degenerative conditions or more importantly live a less happy, content life. It's not like it's all going so damn well on the existing advice now is it? Whoever wrote the Eat Well crap should be ashamed of themselves and I'm pleased to see comments posted under their advice saying as much. Worse yet though, I've met doctors who are the perfect reflection of this advice and attitude too. They don't get it. They don't get that this advice has failed and it has failed because it is wrong and does not suit many, many people.

If you're physically very active you need a diet to fuel that. If you are someone who doesn't get a high insulin response when you eat carbs – and I've read that up to 25 per cent of people are made that way – then the negative effects of eating a lot of carbs, especially weight gain, may not affect you as much, though plenty of researchers believe that too much sugar in your blood provokes degenerative diseases even if you don't put weight on.

It seems eminently sensible to me that a diet high in starchy bulk was established when we lived very different, physically demanding lives, like my grandparents did. Foods such as potatoes and bread were cheap for the poor to fill up on when few other options were available. It was also a diet which, though high in starchy foods, had little or no processed food either and often little sugar. In other words, the context within which it was eaten was very different to today. It is the unique modern combination of high-carb foods, processed foods, high sugars, sweeteners and high fructose corn syrups along with highly processed vegetable oils that provide the witches' brew that has destroyed so many people's health.

So why continue to eat so many carbs? I'd argue from my own experience that there's a far more natural way to eat.

It's not a licence to throw a pint of cream, two kilos of bacon and twenty-four eggs down your throat every day, which some seemed to think it was, especially stateside. God love the Yanks who are professionally dedicated to over-eating no matter what. You can abuse even the best ideas if you try hard enough but it shouldn't be judged by that. Just because many of us have the resources and opportunity to gorge ourselves twenty-four hours a day doesn't mean we should or that we don't need to observe some degree of discipline in our lives.

What I've found is that a higher-fat and lower-carbohydrate diet has remarkably moderated the way I eat and has imposed a natural discipline driven by lower levels of hunger and greater satiation when I do eat. If I'd followed the doctors' and government advice and ate their healthy diet, this simply wouldn't be the case. My only regret, and it is a deep, bitter regret, is that I didn't look for this solution earlier in life and stopped years of ill-health and of dragging a big fat arse around with me.

WHAT IS AND WHAT
SHOULD NEVER BE

I used to be an argumentative sod. I was once thrown out of someone's house (and consequently spent a freezing night in King's Cross station) for furiously arguing that Bob Seger (with or without The Silver Bullet Band) was not just musically better than the newly fashionable Depeche Mode but was actually both morally and spiritually superior. To my 19-year-old mind, Seger's mid-west rock 'n' roll had more grit and integrity than such lightweight Essex pop mincings. Obviously, this is nonsense. You can't make objective arguments about subjective things. You can't make someone feel what you feel about music. But this did not stop me trying with great gusto.

Today I tend to look for the things that unite us rather than divide us but I'd still never listen to early 1980s Depeche Mode, obviously. So in that spirit, I've searched for something that unites all sides of the food divide. We're a long way into *The Meat Fix* and there's been precious little unity of opinion but there is one food on which everyone is agreed: sweet, sweet sugar.

There's nobody out there saying eating sugar is going to give you a long, healthy, cool life. I've yet to find a loopy diet based on eating only sugar, and there's always a loopy diet where you eat just one thing for a week and lose a stone a day, or whatever. Not even the woo-woo crazy people have crossed the sugar rubicon and advocated it as a health food, even though you will find sugar in health food shops – but only brown sugar or raw sugar, as though that makes a difference to anything other than flavour. It sometimes seems anything brown can make it onto the health food store shelves.

Mind you, there are some sugary things which are definitely more hip than others. Rock up at your local health food store and you'll see something called agave syrup on the shelves. This is derived from the agave cacti. Cool, like Tequila, huh? It's a traditional Mexican sweetener and is as sugary as you'd like. It might seem more funky than eating white sugar derived from sugar beets grown under the grey clouds of England, but it is nonetheless sugar and it acts in the same way in your body as regular sugar does. It ain't a healthy version of sugar. Nor is Maple syrup, though it is bloody delicious and compulsive eating.

So at least we can all agree on sugar being bad for you. But from there on, the unity begins to fall apart.

The official advice from the NHS says, 'Many foods that contain added sugars also contain lots of calories, so eating these foods often can contribute to you becoming overweight.'

Well, duh. But hold on, if sugar makes you fat, sugary fruit will make you fat and they don't recommend cutting down on that because Fruit Is Good For You. This is a mantra we must not question.

The long-held traditional view is that sugar pretty much stops at the white stuff in your coffee and cakes. In reality, sugar, in the form of fructose, is in fruits and starchy vegetables too and, as many observers have pointed out, our bodies don't really use those sugars any different to how it uses table sugar. It just takes a slightly different length of time to arrive in your blood as glucose.

The bottom line is if you stuff a spoon of white refined sugar in your mouth, the process isn't much different to putting a banana or a potato in there, except table sugar is actually all sucrose. It all ends up as glucose and it all has to be dealt with by your insulin. My poor insulin, it must have been knackered with all the work I gave it eating so many carbs.

Healthy eating advice doesn't seem to recognise this similarity at all. It seems to want to keep everything in separate departments and never the twain shall meet. The fact is, eating starchy foods, high sugar fruits and especially drinking fruit juice, delivers loads of sugar into your body just as eating loads of granulated sugar does.

We've been sold fruit as a super-healthy thing and it's easy to see why, but that's no reason to go mental and eat your body weight in fruit every day. I used to have five-fruit breakfasts at one point. I thought I was super, super healthy in doing so. Wrong again sucker.

However, at least there are nutrients in fruit, which can't be said of sugar. Clearly, we've gone a bit mad for the white stuff – Americans eat an average of 175lbs of sugar a year! Given that surely some eat less than that, plenty must be eating over 300lbs a year or even more. Good grief. I wouldn't mind betting the UK isn't far behind in this level of consumption. I reckon for most of my first eighteen years of life I ate sugar every single day, being a voracious consumer of cheap sweets. Everything from Fruit Salad and Black Jacks at four for a halfpenny (yes I'm old enough to remember halfpenny's, though not farthings which to you young bucks was one quarter of a penny) to white chocolate mice and fizzy Love Hearts. I'm sure it's just the same for kids today. The difference is, the only thing our parents worried about was rampant tooth decay, whereas nowadays having a bloater child with diabetes by age twelve is a major consideration. Most of us didn't seem to get fat on sugar; maybe we ate less or just as likely we ate it in a different overall food context. Maybe we were also more active each day.

When you roll together our sugar consumption with our fruit and carb consumption, it means our blood sugar is forever on a roller-coaster, spiking after eating and then crashing an hour or two later only then to be raised hugely again by sugary snacks. This just wears you out. I found it bloody exhausting and as I got older it only worked as a lifestyle by endless self-medication: more carbs or sugar or alcohol brought me up again after a crash.

These days I don't eat any sugar at all and rarely eat sugary fruits tending to stick to berries instead. Result? Even moods, no headaches and good levels of energy evenly spread throughout the day. It's a huge change.

Mind you, as bad as sugar might be, arguably worse are artificial sweeteners. You'll find no advice at all about these things from your government or your doctor. Indeed, you could say that the official healthy eating advice of eating less sugar is driving people into the arms of the artificial sweetener business and not without consequence.

Artificial sweeteners are usually aspartame, sucralose, neotame, acesulfame potassium and saccharin. Lovely. What says tasty treat more than acesulfame potassium or neotame? I like neowild myself. Sweeteners are added to many foods but especially to fizzy pop. It's even added to the non-diet varieties.

When I was a kid, a lorry would come around the streets

carrying crates of pop for sale. 'The Pop Man' was greeted like the Pied Piper by herds of thirsty children clutching a two-bob bit given to them by their mam. The pop came in heavy glass bottles with a black rubber bung as a stopper. This sounds like a bucolic scene from the 1920s doesn't it?

Getting a bottle of pop was actually a real treat, not an everyday event in the 1960s. A bottle of something comparatively exotic such as cream soda, which was for some reason dyed bright green, was like drinking nectar from the slipper of an angel.

As the 1970s progressed, cans of pop became more ubiquitous. Not just Coke and Pepsi but Fanta, Tizer and Cresta. Around the mid 1970s I remember Tab Cola being sold in my local newsagent. It was advertised as a 'diet' cola and had just one calorie. It was very popular with girls right away but my recollection is of it tasting like a watery cough medicine which left your throat slightly sore and a strange bitter flavour on your tongue. Much like Watneys Red Barrel, a heinous 1970s chemical beer of the era.

Diet sodas had been around since the 1950s and early 1960s but probably didn't make it to these shores in any amount until the early 1970s. Tab was made by Coca-Cola and that weird taste was saccharin, later banned as potentially carcinogenic, largely because rats developed bladder cancer when fed it. Poor ratty. What have they done to you, lad? Surely though, rats are not made physiologically to handle drinking coke and are bound to go wrong on it. It's probably the equivalent of giving us a bleach and Toilet Duck cocktail. Mmm ... Toilet Duck.

This shocking discovery didn't mean saccharin was banned, oh no, it just had to be put on labels so you knew it was in there, just in case you wanted your pet rat to get bladder cancer. Later, it turned out that the rat's cancer wasn't caused by saccharin, which all goes to prove the limited use of testing food on rats. So now you don't even need to warn people it's in your soda – presumably your bladder is safe.

While almost all other foodstuffs are keen to shout at us that they have 'no artificial flavourings or colours' especially when it comes to food that kids like because they don't want parents feeling guilty about feeding them chemically enhanced rubbish, when it comes to soda drinks no one seems to give a toss. Whack in as much artificial sweetener as you want fella because hey, it's not sugar, so it must be more healthy, right? Err … no and did you know your brain is leaking out of your eyes and your head is on fire? The healthy eating advice is rightly anti sugar but it should be every bit as anti artificial sweeteners.

Rather than artificial sweeteners being more slimming than sugar, there's now some evidence that, ironically, drinking more diet soda makes you more likely to get fat.

Honestly, this is the bizarro world you are taking part in if you drink this stuff. Let's just restate this for clarity, the diet soda the weight conscious people buy with their 12-inch pizza to offset the high-calorie guilt, might be making some people fatter.

This from Tara Parker-Pope of the *Wall Street Journal* in July 2007:

'There have been suggestions in the literature that diet soda may not be innocuous,' says Vasan S. Ramachandran, associate professor at the Boston University School of Medicine and senior investigator on the study. 'We have explanations that we offer as theories, but we need additional research.'

The research was immediately criticised by the soft-drink industry and some nutrition researchers. 'There is no plausible physiological mechanism to explain this and causes me to question the accuracy of the methodologies used in this study,' says Dean Ornish [sounds like a character in Kerouac's *On The Road* doesn't he?], clinical professor of medicine at the University of California, San Francisco, and chairman of the PepsiCo Health & Wellness Advisory Board.

The new report from the Framingham study compared soft-drink consumption among nearly 9,000 middle-aged men and women. Overall, soda drinkers were at 48 per cent higher risk for metabolic syndrome, a collection of health problems including being overweight, and having blood-sugar levels signalling diabetes risk. The risks of metabolic syndrome were about the same whether the soft drink was sugared or sugar-free. The study authors noted that the research doesn't prove sodas cause health problems.

The American Beverage Association, which represents soft-drink companies, said it is 'scientifically implausible' to suggest diet drinks could cause weight gain or elevated blood pressure. 'All of our industry's beverages ... can be part of a healthy way of life when consumed in moderation,' said ABA President Susan K. Neely in a statement.

But the data on diet soda has been mixed. One previous study showed a link between diet-soda consumption and weight gain in boys. Some research has suggested that artificial sweeteners may 'condition' diet-soda drinkers to develop a preference for sweet, higher-calorie foods. Other studies have questioned whether the caramel content of both regular and diet soft drinks may play a role in insulin resistance.

Nutritionists say the study should be a wake-up call for soda drinkers, noting that a zero-calorie beverage can't undo the damage of an unhealthy diet.

Now I don't want to be alarmist about these sweeteners but frankly, you might as well put a bit of heroin in your kid's coke, at least it would keep them quiet for a while and they might dump their hideous dance music downloads and buy Velvet Underground albums instead. Which would be huge progress, by the way. Ok, I'm joking, don't go making your Nicholson Says Put Our Kids On Heroin headlines. Mind you, my mam used to give me half of a small barbituate tablet to make me relax and go to sleep when I was an anxious young boy. Maybe this explains my fondness for The Velvet Underground.

But even if you don't want to believe that artificial sweeteners make you fatter, there are other, perhaps even more troubling issues. Some researchers reckon aspartame sweeteners, along with additives such as MSG, hydrolyzed vegetable protein and other flavour enhancers are excito-toxins that fry your brain. 'Brain frying' is in all the medical dictionaries, I think you'll find.

One of these is a dude called Russell L. Blaylock, MD who has researched its effects in detail in his tome, *Excitoxins: The Taste That Kills*:

> There are a growing number of clinicians and basic scientists who are convinced that excitotoxins play a critical role in the development of several neurological disorders, including migraines, seizures, infections, abnormal neural development, certain endocrine disorders, specific types of obesity, and especially the neurodegenerative diseases; a group of diseases which includes: ALS, Parkinson's disease, Alzheimer's disease, Huntington's disease, and olivopontocerebellar degeneration.

And you know how bad olivopontocerebellar degeneration is. No, neither do I but it sounds like it'd put a cramp in your weekend, doesn't it?

Blaylock goes on to say:

> An enormous amount of both clinical and experimental evidence has accumulated over the past decade supporting this basic premise. Yet, the FDA (America's food and drug administration) still refuses to recognise the immediate and long term danger to the public caused by the practice of allowing various excitotoxins to be added to the food supply, such as MSG, hydrolyzed vegetable protein, and aspartame.

Well it's such a massive business isn't it? No government is going to take on that kind of financial and cultural muscle. Coca-Cola is the imperialist outrider for American culture, found in even the most distant and obscure corners of the earth. Are you going to tell them they're messing with our brains? Well Blaylock is. He points out that the amount of these neurotoxins added to our food has increased enormously since their first introduction. Since 1948 the amount of MSG added to foods has doubled every decade. By 1972, 262,000 metric tons were being added to foods. Over 800 million pounds of aspartame have been consumed in various products since it was first approved. That is one big heap of artificialness!

Here's the revolutionary thought: we could, probably within a few weeks, put the producers of them out of business by, gulp, not eating them! Shock. Same goes for Coca-Cola et al. We all just stop. Simple. Or so you'd think. It will never happen because too many are enslaved to them but the public en masse must be made aware that these excitotoxins are not present in just a few foods but rather in almost all processed foods. In many cases they are being added in disguised forms, such as natural flavouring, spices, yeast extract, textured protein and soy protein extract. We've all seen TV programmes about kids who live on junk food and are hyper, destructive, tearful and generally crazed. And we've seen how they calm down when fed unadulterated, wholesome food. This must be because of all those sweeteners and flavourings in the processed food. And if it affects kids, why wouldn't it affect adults too?

Now if I'm going to have my brain fried, I'd at least like a few colourful hallucinations while listening to 'Dark Star' by the Grateful Dead. Having a life-altering psychedelic experience is at least a good trade off against the loss of brain cells, in a way that necking some sweet drink just isn't.

Sweeteners are rightly controversial but are a huge business and can afford lots of lawyers to defend themselves against accusations that their products are harmful. The artificial sweetener industry is reported as being worth anywhere between $700 million and $1 billion per year or more. Surprising then that they have never sued Blaylock nor threatened to. He feels this is because he knows too much and they don't want his research being brought into the open. It's certainly plausible.

It's my view that any healthy eating advice from your doctor or the NHS should be addressing these issues. Sweeteners are potentially major influences over the health of the population but warnings are utterly ignored in favour of telling us not to eat full-cream milk. Well fucking done.

Yes the evidence about artificial sweeteners is controversial and not unanimously agreed upon, but then that is true for everything the health police push as unequivocal advice. And if you stop and think about it, is it really a good idea to put these chemicals into our bodies in such large and frequent amounts? Given the increase in such disorders in kids as autism and ADD as well as the widespread problems with depression, you have to wonder if these very modern witches' brews are now at least in the mix when it comes to their causation.

However, while many of us have always had an intuitive notion that anything with 'artificial' in front of it is probably not as good for us, at least not as good as *not* consuming it, good, honest, old-fashioned salt is at least a natural thing. There is, remarkably, an artificial salt, or at least a low sodium one. Of course there is, there's always a pervy version of something perfectly natural. But somehow, the low-salt salt doesn't seem to have caught on like Diet Coke.

But it exists because salt is bad for you too, you know. Oh yes, you know it, I know it. We all know it. We're not sure how or why we know it or why it's so bad but you'll see 'reduced salt' options on plenty of products in your supermarket.

The Blood Pressure Association says this about the salty stuff:

> The amount of salt you eat has a direct effect on your blood pressure. Salt makes your body hold on to water. If you eat too much salt, the extra water stored in your body raises your blood pressure. So, the more salt you eat, the higher your blood pressure. The higher your blood pressure, the greater the strain on your heart, arteries, kidneys and brain. This can lead to heart attacks, strokes, dementia and kidney disease.

Yikes. Dementia. Salty lunatics! Who doesn't know someone driven mad by salt? Seriously, though, this is about as scary as you can get. Given the amount of salt eaten, if this is true, it's amazing anyone is left standing or sane in Western Europe or indeed in almost all other parts of the world.

Salt has been so important to humanity that people have fought wars over it and founded ports specifically to export it. France even taxed it from the Middle Ages onwards and only finally repealed this in 1945, presumably to reward their people's war effort.

Humans of all races and societies from the dawn of time have, perhaps appropriately enough, been mad for salt. Of course, the good old NHS Eat Well website has plenty of warnings about the stuff. It doesn't care about aspartame frying your brain, no, no no, but in 'Salt: The Facts' it announces with more certainty than it really should,

> Many of us in the UK eat too much salt. Too much salt can raise your blood pressure, which puts you at increased risk of health problems such as heart disease and stroke.

It continues to belch in a salty cloud of hot air,

> Other foods, such as bread and breakfast cereals, can contribute a lot of salt to our diet. But that's not because these foods are always high in salt: it's because we eat a lot of them.

Whoa whoa, hold on there. 'We eat a lot of them.' Yes, because you tell us to. You say to base our diet on starchy foods and grains, including bread and breakfast cereals which come with lots of added salt, so don't be surprised if people buy them. It's enough to make you punch your computer.

I was always very salt conscious; you learned to be early on in the wholefood, hippy world of eating. It was almost a given that you were careful how much you added to your meals. I wasn't even that certain as to why I was being careful with it but I was sure there must have been a good, well-proven reason.

By now you will not be surprised to learn that if it's on the NHS healthy eating website list of foods to be worried about, many people think this is scaremongering nonsense. The idea that salt is bad for all of us is a tad contentious to say the least, indeed, it is in all likelihood for most people utter, utter bollocks.

You can definitely poison yourself with salt as you can with almost anything. A few tablespoons a day might not be especially efficacious, not unless you're trying to preserve yourself from the inside out. But officially we're not supposed to have more than a teaspoon's worth a day, about 6 grams. Given the prevalence of salt in processed food, this is probably exceeded by almost everyone every day.

Michael Alderman who is President of the American Society of Hypertension (I bet their Christmas parties are just fantastic), Department of Epidemiology and Social Medicine, Albert Einstein College of Medicine, wrote in 1997:

> Public health recommendations must be based on proof of safety and benefit. Even if a low sodium diet could lower the blood pressure of most people (probably not true) and both the diet and the change in blood pressure could be sustained (not established), this alone would not justify a recommendation to reduce sodium intake.

So you've been cutting back for no reason at all. It doesn't stop there. Earlier, a 2011 study, which followed 3,681 healthy European men and women aged sixty or younger for about eight years, also found that above-average salt intake did not appear to increase the danger of developing high blood pressure. The report, which was published in the Journal of the American Medical Association, was released just three months after the US government launched a public health campaign urging restaurants and food manufacturers to cut down on their use of salt. Oops. That was a bit off message.

Sodium was measured in the urine of those taking part, at the beginning and end of the study (always a nice job first thing in the morning after you've been out on the town!).

Little more than 6 per cent of the participants suffered a heart attack, a stroke or some other cardiovascular emergency during the eight years. About a third of these were fatal. Those who consumed the least salt had a 56 per cent higher risk of death from a heart attack or stroke compared with those who consumed the most!

This was even after obesity, cholesterol levels, smoking, diabetes and other risk factors were taken into account. There were fifty deaths in the third of participants with the lowest salt consumption, twenty-four in the third with medium intake and just ten deaths in those with the highest salt levels.

Lead researcher Jan Staessen, head of the hypertension laboratory at the University of Leuven, in Belgium, said: 'Our findings do not support a generalised reduction of salt intake in the population.'

The scientists couldn't really explain their results, but speculated that low levels of salt in the body could cause more stress in the nervous system, decrease sensitivity to insulin and affect hormones that control blood pressure and sodium absorption. But they stressed that those with high blood pressure – who were not included in the study – should still stick to a low-salt diet.

While this is just one study, and its methodology has been questioned (methodologies are always questioned; if you want to discredit anything, question its methodologies. I think this is because the word methodologies sounds quite technical and if you can drop it into a sentence casually it sounds like you must know what you're talking about), it has long been said that salt is no risk to anyone who hasn't had a heart attack or doesn't have elevated blood pressure and it won't cause those things to happen in the bodies of healthy people if you eat it in anything like the normal amount of up to 15–16g a day. Given most salt consumed in the west is as a part of processed food and not added at the table, I think I'd be less inclined to blame salt per se for high blood pressure. (Though what is high blood pressure is actually a bone of contention in itself. The level said to be high has been lowered over the years and thus allowed more hypertension drugs to be prescribed just as it has been with cholesterol figures. Follow the money. It'd make more sense to look at how it works as a part of a diet that is high in processed food and sugar, wouldn't it? What's that you say? There's no money for the drug companies in that? Don't be so cynical.)

Me, I only use Maldon sea salt because it's a lot more salty in flavour and because I'm a food ponce. My blood pressure isn't high and doesn't seem affected by my salt intake at all. In fact, I've tried making it higher by making all my food much more salty for a week but it didn't work. It made no difference. The resting rate was still always a couple of beats either side of 114/75.

Dawn has low blood pressure and eats up to 10g of salt per day. No effect at all. Hardly a scientific experiment, I'll grant you but we like playing with our blood pressure monitor. Oh yes, there's nothing like measuring your postural hypotension if you want to get the party started. Groovy.

Salt is just one more thing to make you paranoid if you're so inclined. I'd be more worried about worrying about salt than about actually eating salt – all that worry is bound to give you hypertension.

This is where we are in the twenty-first century, driven to distraction, worried by food and by what it's doing to us. This is what the healthy eating propagandists have made us.

And while we're talking about making the public worried, let's have a look at another state-sponsored nannying scheme, the nonsense that is the 'five-fruit-and-veg-a-day' campaign. As a healthy-eating vegetarian, if there was one thing that I thought made me super-healthy it was eating up to fifteen portions of fruit and veg a day. My vegetable consumption was huge. I was a holy man when it came to vegetables.

Until I did some research, like you, I'm sure, I assumed five fruit and veg a day was based on some kind of hard science but it isn't really. It's just made up. Honestly. This subject was even mentioned recently on an edition of *QI*: five was merely as much as they thought the British public would in their wildest dreams manage to eat, so they plumped for that as a target. There's no specific science to justify five a day.

In some parts of Europe the recommendation is to eat more than five vegetables per day. In America it includes potatoes, over here it doesn't. Some include tinned fruit and vegetables others do not. The portion sizes vary from country to country too. There's nothing rationalised or standardised about it. If you eat four portions there is no estimated or measured difference over and above eating say five, six or ten. This is because five is an arbitrary amount.

It seems to be based on some studies that showed that people who ate more fruit and veg suffered from less heart attacks, stroke and cancer. Great. After all, there's no pain in having to eat vegetables, not unless you're Scottish anyway.

However, there are questions as to the validity of such assumed connection between fruit and veg consumption and better health. People who eat more fruit and veg might also have other lifestyle factors in their favour. They may do more exercise, smoke less or not stab themselves in the face with a compass as much, who knows?

Some of the more alternative researchers have pointed to

the Eskimos for evidence of how humans can survive very well without any fruit and vegetables. Apparently Eskimos lived for millennia off nothing but seal blubber and fish and never got any modern western diseases.

Given their lives were lived in the icy wastes of the North Pole, I'd have thought that was a bit of a bummer really. Surely the quicker death comes, the less time you've got to spend gazing out over featureless frozen landscapes or wrestling polar bears. Anyway, this might be a lifestyle specific to them, which they uniquely evolved to survive their environment due to the lack of a decent public transport system to take them south to warmer regions – surely a better option.

Even if this is all true, I'm not sure that would necessarily be appropriate to people who live in, say, Hartlepool in the twenty-first century, not least because you can't buy seal blubber in Hartlepool, even though it's not without its featureless icy wastelands.

The idea behind the five-a-day campaign is obviously to give people some sort of focus for getting more fruit and vegetables into them and that's not so evil, I suppose, but it treats all fruit and veg as though it's equally as good for you and that five of anything is desirable. Well, there's nothing comparable between say celery and an avocado. One is rich in nutrition, the other much less so. And, as we know, eating very sugary fruit can spike your insulin and cause you to gain weight or at least not lose it.

Eating an apple, an orange, a banana, a couple of carrots and a sweet potato has an entirely different nutritional composition to say, an onion, celery, cabbage, peas and green beans, and would be digested quite differently. It's not explained why it doesn't matter which veg you eat, only that you should eat five or more.

A big study called Cardio 2000 came to this conclusion,

Our findings support that even low consumption of fruits and vegetables (1–2 servings per week) is associated with about 45 per cent lower coronary risk. Consumption of two or more servings per week is associated with about 70 per cent reduction in relative risk.

Sir Charles George, medical director of the British Heart Foundation, said of these results 'There is some argument about how much you need – I think five may be an arbitrary figure.'

The Harvard School of Public Health did a study in 2004 of over 100,000 people and concluded that

Increased fruit and vegetable consumption was associated with a modest although not statistically significant reduction in the development of major chronic disease.

Such benefits they did discover appeared to be mainly for cardiovascular disease and not for cancer. They finally 'fessed up and said,

Consumption of five or more servings of fruits and vegetables has been recommended but the protective effect of fruit and vegetable intake may have been overstated.

And there we were thinking that it was some sort of gospel truth. No one really thinks that eating fruit and veg is bad for you. But the holy status given to five a day is somewhat controversial. More isn't always better. More might be OK but not essential for a long happy life and quite probably not worth fretting so much about.

It's certainly true that most vegetables are simply not that nutritious when compared to animal products and thus, contribute much less to our diet. The obsession with fruit and vegetables is an over-focus on foods which give us little in return and perhaps not even that much protection against disease.

Nutritionist and author Zoe Harcombe in her book *The Obesity Epidemic* looked into this and discovered a large study that examined half a million people over eight years and reported that fruit and vegetables offered no protection against breast, prostate, bowel, lung or any other kind of tumour. In fact, those eating the most fruit and veg showed no difference in cancer risk compared with those eating the least. Blimey.

She goes on to say that fruit and veg are pretty useless, nutritionally.

There are thirteen vitamins and fruit is good for one of them: vitamin C. Vegetables offer some vitamins – vitamin C and the vegetable form of the fat-soluble vitamin A and vitamin K1 – but your body will be able to absorb these only if you add some fat, such as butter or olive oil. The useful forms of A and K – retinol and K2 respectively – are found only in animal foods. As for minerals, there are sixteen and fruit is good for one of them, potassium, which is not a substance we are often short of, as it is found in water. Vegetables can be OK for iron and calcium but the vitamins and minerals in animal foods (meat, fish, eggs and dairy products) beat those in fruit and vegetables hands down. There is far more vitamin A in liver than in an apple, for instance ... the five-a-day idea started as a marketing campaign dreamt up by around twenty fruit and veg companies and the US National Cancer Institute at a meeting in California in 1991. And it's been remarkably successful.

This doesn't strike me as a case for not eating vegetables so much as for not over-stating how magnificent they are for your good health. I ate up to fifteen portions of fruit and veg most days for over twenty years and it didn't do me much good. It might have been worse if I hadn't eaten them I suppose; it could also have been better. I'll never know. Certainly our sewerage pipe would not have had so much wear and tear.

The five-a-day campaign has elevated veg to an almost mythic status. As long as you eat them, everything else will be OK. That's just way too simplistic and over-stated. If you've eaten four before midnight and then have an apple after midnight does that count towards that day's total or the next? Once you set a defined amount, it suggests specific results as a consequence of eating that defined amount and yet there are no definable specific results available.

There is also growing concern that fruit and veg has less nutrition than it did say fifty years ago because the soil it grows in has been denuded of nutrients through over production and reliance on artificial fertilisers. A landmark study on the topic by Donald Davis and his team of researchers from the University of Texas was published in December 2004 in the *Journal of the American College of Nutrition*. They studied US Department of Agriculture nutritional data from both 1950 and 1999 for forty-three different vegetables and fruits, finding 'reliable declines' in the amount of protein, calcium, phosphorus, iron, riboflavin (vitamin B2) and vitamin C over the past half century. Davis put this down to declining nutritional content to the preponderance of agricultural practices designed to improve size, growth rate and pest resistance.

I guess it all depends what you compare vegetables to as a valuable food stuff. As Zoe Harcombe points out, you can get more nutrition more easily from eggs, meat or fish. But compared to a diet of highly processed food which is high in sugar and vegetable fat, the veg is looking pretty good. It's all relative.

When my head feels like it's going to explode with all these contradictions, as ever, I go back to how my grandparents ate for some sanity and sense on all these issues.

They ploughed through large amounts of brassicas: cabbages, sprouts, broccoli, cauliflowers, plenty of carrots and turnip and swede, marrows, leeks, onions and green beans. In summer they'd major on tomatoes, cucumber, radishes, celery and lettuce. They didn't need telling that it was good for them, they knew it was. No meal came without a heap of veg. All of these were either home grown, locally grown or at least came from the UK and were grown in season, not imported from elsewhere in the world. I do wonder if we're not genetically programmed to eat food in season and eating it out of season freaks our bodies out somehow. We could never eat fruit and veg out of season until relatively recently.

The grandparents certainly ate them all up and considered it to be a sin if us kids didn't do likewise. Leaving your sprouts wasn't just frowned upon, it was simply not allowed. You sat there until you ate them, even crying and saying you felt sick made no difference. 'Get them ate.' This may have been a cruel streak in them or just good common sense. The legacy of this discipline meant in adult life I never disliked any vegetable or fruit and even now feel almost morally obliged to eat everything on my plate.

Seeing people in restaurants picking at their food, separating out the celery or peas or radishes or whatever the hell it is that they think they don't like just drives me nuts. I turn into my gran, thinking aggressively to myself 'get it bloody eaten and stop pushing it around your plate, it's not going to go away'. Being so fussy seems to me, like it did to them, just massively bourgeois and self indulgent.

As for too much salt giving you a heart-attack, they'd have laughed in mockery at that. I can just hear Fred, 'Whoever told you that needs to take a look at 'imself. If that was true, we'd all be dead!'

Artificial sweeteners would have been thrown out for being fancy, modern and 'made in a bloody factory some-where', which was OK if it was a big metal machine but not OK if it was food.

So to sum up, your healthy eating advice probably over-rates fruit and veg, worries too much about salt, not enough about artificial sweeteners or about some forms of sugar. Not a good record. No surprise then that we have rising obesity and depression rates.

OK, let's just pause and look back over all of this. We have been told how to eat for the last thirty years to be healthy: low in animal fat and high in starches, fruit, vegetables and wholegrains. In that thirty years obesity has gone up exponentially as have all manner of other lifestyle diseases. Throughout that whole period there were dissenting voices that said this was a crazy departure from what humans had evolved to eat and what they had always thrived on.

Throughout this time there has been a boom in processed food and along with this a huge increase in artificial sweet-eners and flavourings such as aspartame, MSG, hydrolyzed vegetable protein and many others. Use of all vegetable oils, especially soya oil has expanded enormously and low-fat spreads and skimmed milk have become entirely normal, regular purchases. Soya and wheat feature in ever expanding lists of products. A new type of wheat has been developed at a time when gluten intolerance has grown enormously.

The healthy eating advice from doctors and governments has not sought to address any of these issues. They have stuck to their low-fat and high-carb, wholegrain message as the health of the west slowly falls apart. They must be so proud.

Here's the NHS statistics on obesity, physical activity and diet, reported in 2011:

In 2009, almost a quarter of adults (22 per cent of men and 24 per cent of women) were obese, and 66 per cent of men and 57 per cent of women were overweight including obese.

However, the same report says in 2008 that 39 per cent of men and 29 per cent of women aged sixteen and over met the then government's recommendations for physical activity, compared with 32 per cent and 21 per cent respectively in 1997. So people are getting more physically active.

By 2015, the NHS figures predict that 36 per cent of males and 28 per cent of females (aged between twenty-one and sixty) will be obese. By 2025 it is estimated that 47 per cent of men and 36 per cent of women will be obese. A 2009 Health and Safety Executive report shows that around three in ten children aged two to fifteen were classed as either overweight or obese.

However, as Hannah Sutter says in her book *Big Fat Lies*, our calorie intake has dropped by 20 per cent since 1974 and we have actually increased our fruit and veg intake by 20 per cent in the same period, though this has begun to decrease with the recession. We are now doing more exercise – 25 per cent more than we did in 1997. We are also following government advice and eating much less saturated animal fat, primarily through the growth in sales of margarine and low-fat spreads, skimmed milk and through use of vegetable oils rather than animal fat in most processed foods.

Consumption of sugar is reported at 12.5 per cent of energy consumed, which sounds high, however the NHS recommends it be just 1.5 per cent less at 11 per cent, which is surely still too high.

While it's clear from all the surveys done that people are increasingly following the guidelines they're being given, it's really not making any great difference to the health of the nation. While the authorities can argue that people just need to follow them to a greater extent and for longer, an equally, if not more, plausible view is that the recommendations simply don't work for a lot of people and indeed make things worse for many. Healthy eating, for those people, just like for me, simply isn't healthy. Either that, or at a time of unprecedented food wealth and availability, over-consumption is just too easy to do.

It would be a huge *volte face* for everyone to admit these mistakes and inevitably it would be greeted with howls of 'you don't know what you're doing' from the general public, who are already at the end of their tether when it comes to be being told how to eat.

Indeed, when you read the NHS literature on diet and lifestyle the impression you get is of a confused and slightly desperate organisation, thrashing around in the dark trying to draw a straight line between people's diseases and their lifestyles. But it is a straight line which often resolutely refuses to be drawn. For example their stats show that while being overweight increases your likelihood of having high blood pressure, the majority of obese and morbidly obese men don't actually have high blood pressure.

It's like the stats on heart attacks: people with low cholesterol have them just as much as high, even more perhaps. Similarly we all know people who eat huge amounts of food and don't ever put a pound in weight on.

The human body is such a hard-to-predict beast and seems to steadfastly refuse to do the same thing from person to person. This is simply self-evident and bearing it in mind, surely a more wide-ranging and flexible approach to dietary recommendations would at least be an intelligent approach. To present and account for other ways to eat and live would at least give people some tools for looking at what really suits them. Not to do so is simply negligent and given these circumstances it is both highly understandable and desirable that people follow different paths when they find those recommended don't work or make things much worse.

The thought that I'd still be suffering from chronic IBS, still be fat and unhealthy if I had believed that no cholesterol, low fat, high carbs was the healthy diet is what drove me to spend a year of my life writing this book. It haunts me that health and well-being were so close, so within reach and yet so elusive. I shouldn't feel bitter, I should just let it go but I can't. I'm furious at myself for being so stubborn but I'm also furious at the medical people and official eating advice for their utter, utter failure to help in any way at all.

I think by and large we used to know how to eat. My grandparents' generation certainly did. They ate a diet that suited their way of life, just as many did in that time. That sensibility seems to have been extinguished by the 1980s. Today, we're all so very fucked up about food. We need to get back to what we used to know, get back to eating wholesome, homemade food, and we need to eat a diet that suits us and our lives personally even if it's not what the doctor ordered.

LIFE IS A CARNIVAL, BELIEVE IT OR NOT

I was talking to an old friend about how I'd given up being that old vegetarian type dude, that I'd put away my orange robes, red lentils and George Harrison albums, especially the 1980s stuff, which is pretty awful anyway. How I'd not just embraced a whole new way of life but had gripped it firmly by the neck, the way a bouncer grabs you outside a nightclub when you step over the roped off area without permission, and that I wasn't about to let go.

As we talked, he kept referring to this change of circumstances as my 'lifestyle' as though it was a kind of bullet-pointed programme that could be followed, a laminated 'how-to' guide. That there were rules to be followed and things that were 'allowed' and 'banned'.

Well saddle up the Palomino Tonto because that really ain't me and how I now eat isn't anything special nor is it especially original. It's not like I live on deep-fried mice rolled in opium. It certainly isn't something I have invented. Sure, it's not 'normal' in that the majority of people don't eat this way, but when you call something a lifestyle it sounds more grand than it actually feels when you get up in a morning and stare out at the rain and wonder what another day of consciousness will bring.

Rather, I reckon it's quite a modest way to go through life. Very down to earth and practical. You might even call it natural, though I know that word, above all others when it comes to food, is the most used and abused. When I hear it called a lifestyle it makes it seem harder, bigger and more difficult to do, when it's really piss easy. Creating a lifestyle is for Californian women called Sunflower or for dudes with better abs than mine.

Besides, when people do create such regimes they are always keen to sell it as though it is a magical answer to everyone's problems; the ultimate solution. No self-doubt. Look at any self-appointed food guru's books or websites and you won't find any uncertainty, or usually any mention of other ways of life or diets. It's their way or the highway.

Now call me flaky if you want but my whole approach these days isn't about that. It's about finding what really suits you personally. That's who really matters after all, right? It's about liberating yourself from the dictat of conventional wisdom on healthy eating, sticking it to the man and about finding your own, what the Grateful Dead called a golden road to devotion, but what I shall call ... errr ... path.

If there's one over-riding message to take away from all of this it is that the one-size fits all healthy eating advice is ridiculous and plainly does not apply to, or suit, most people. How could it? We're all different creatures. I mean, OK, we're the same species, though I do wonder sometimes, y'know, some people look like they grew under a rock. But there the similarities end. If we were all the same we'd all die at the same time from the same disease, which would be handy and very convenient for all concerned. You could time yourself down to expiry on a specially made Death Watch. I digress or as my gran would have said, 'you're talking loud and saying nothing' or was that James Brown?

Clearly, we are all different, both in how we are made genetically but also in our personal food and health histories. We arrive at this point from a myriad of different angles and starting points. So exactly what we will thrive on today and what we won't will inevitably be different from person to person. Differences will be small, vast and everything in between.

However, what I do believe, after all my research and journeys into the sometimes gothic world of alternative healthy eating, is that reducing the amount of carbohydrates you eat, eating plenty of organic, pasture-fed meats and fats and ceasing to eat processed foods would be a good move for many, many people for many, many reasons, not least of which it would lead to a reduction in weight. But also, just as important, an increase in a sense of well-being.

I don't believe anyone thrives on processed food and we will never be all we can be health-wise if it forms a substantial part of our diet. All those contrived soya products wrecked my health. Of course it varies hugely in quality; some processed foods are much better than others. But none of them are better or equal to making meals from scratch from quality ingredients.

This need not be difficult or time consuming. How long does it take to boil an egg, fry a piece of fish or steak? Less time than it takes you to defrost a piece of frozen crap in a microwave that isn't even big enough to fill your belly. Feeding yourself badly in order to save a bit of time makes no sense. By not feeding yourself properly you won't be performing efficiently and will inevitably waste more time on unprofitable, unfocused work than you would have spent on creating a proper meal in the first place. It's a lose-lose situation. Abusing yourself with unwholesome food on the basis that it is occasionally marginally quicker to get it down your meat hole gains you nothing at all. It's important to wake up to this fact. If you don't feed yourself properly, all other bets are off.

I also think this dietary shift has reconnected me with the past, with my food heritage and has disengaged me from the insane modern food world full of lurid advertising and weird ideas about what is and isn't natural. It's allowed me to relax about food. As a vegetarian, I see now that I was uptight about it. Everything was a political statement, everything was another box ticked. Now, having stripped it all back to basics, it feels liberating and it feels good to be part of a more ancient tradition of meat eating. I used to want to be divorced from that tradition; today it feels right to be connected to it.

And if I might indulge in a little bit of cosmic philosophy for a brief moment, I now also feel connected to the wheel of existence, to the circle of life and death from which I was trying to divorce myself as a non-meat eater. This isn't glory in death but an acceptanec of an innate part of being alive. It feels ... what is the word? It feels ... whole.

But of course mostly it just feels brilliant not to be wondering if you're about to shit yourself in public.

The focus of most healthy eating advice is on weight, specifically on losing weight. Mr and Ms Lard Ass is such a literally big presence in our lives that it's hard to ignore. So many degenerative issues are created or aggravated by being overweight. However, not being fat doesn't mean you're well on any level, not physically and certainly not mentally.

Criminally over-looked when it comes to healthy eating advice is how your diet dictates your emotions, your attitudes, your moods, your peace of mind. We are undeniably comprised of what we eat. We know food affects our brain chemistry, no one denies that, but go to a doctor and suggest you are depressed or disturbed because of the food you eat and they're not likely to be sympathetic. They'll pretty quickly issue you with a prescription for strong narcotics to combat your depression without even stopping for a moment to consider if a change of diet could be the solution. I know, I've seen it happen. Yeah, good work, doc. How long were you at university? Not long enough, punk.

This is extraordinarily narrow-minded and quite frankly is not good enough. I don't understand why it happens. I suspect it is primarily because most doctors have no real understanding of diet and nutrition or how it works its magic on us, except for some generalised text book stuff taught to them at college.

It is undoubtedly true that I have undergone a major mental change. No, I wasn't running around the streets with my underpants on my head and a screwdriver in my ear beforehand, but the change has been almost as profound as if I had been.

Emotions, feelings and moods are nebulous things at the best of times; how do you measure, quantify or describe them? There's no wooden ruler you can whip out to measure your feel good factor. However, I know I'm calmer, less volatile, think more clearly, cope with stress much easier, sleep better and am just less prone to fretting about things. Call it an increased sense of well-being. It is as though turbulent waters have become becalmed, as well as a turbulent arse.

How we feel in our heads is such an important part of life. We only seem to address it when things go badly wrong but how we are mentality is the actual reality of our existence. It is how we construct the world around us, how we deal with it and how we appreciate it from hour to hour. While dragging a big belly around with you is a physical manifestation of a health issue, no such symbol shows how we are inside our minds. Unless you've gone proper crazy and start smashing clocks because you think they're listening to you, there is no outward sign of ill-health, yet it is where happiness, sadness, joy and depression lie.

If we sluggishly just get through a day on half power because we are not feeding ourselves properly, then we're not living life to the full, not getting the most out of each day. If a better life is available through your choices of food, why wouldn't you take it and why don't the health professionals pay it any attention whatsoever?

I'll take you through what I do and don't eat and why. Once again, I'm not saying this is the only or the definitive way to eat, only that if it suits me so well then I reckon it might suit you too. Indeed, from what I've read, it is a way of life that many people already follow and feel great on.

Remember though, this isn't like taking magic mushrooms, more's the pity. The positive effects don't kick in half an hour after you've eaten and there shouldn't be any colourful hallucinations either. Do feel free to listen to acid rock and stare at your trousers for several hours though.

The effect of both mental and physical improvement is a steady, gradual one. It may take time to heal and recover from your old diet and lifestyle. While the curing of my IBS was a quick, almost instant sign of how a change of diet was good for me, all the other subsequent benefits have happened over the last year and a half and of course, are continuing to evolve.

By any definition, food is medicine as well as nutrition and pleasure, so remember what the dormouse said: feed your head.

ORGANIC

Whatever you're eating, try and make sure as much of it is organically grown as possible. There's a lot of old cobblers spouted about organically grown food. Some think of it as the holy grail of food; it's like, food grown naturally maaaaaan.

Others think it's just a typically self-obsessed food indulgence of the liberal middle classes who seek to buy stuff which makes them look part of an elite. Many more think it's a rip off and is not any more healthy a choice than the cheaper non-organic stuff and that it doesn't taste any better anyway.

Here's the truth, alright, all of the above can be true. Some do use food as part of their social status and organic works for some people in that context. Sometimes it is no better for you nutritionally than well grown non-organic food. Sometimes it doesn't taste any better, though it usually does. If you grow organically in knackered soil it probably won't be more nutritious than non-organic grown in good soil. And it does attract a premium price, and you might wonder how since less has actually been done to it. And just to confuse matters even more, some organically grown foods are better than other organically grown foods due to better soil, growing conditions or varieties.

I'm not poncy or snobby about organic. The fact is 'conventionally' grown food – I don't know why it's called conventionally grown really because food was grown without artificial fertilisers and pesticides for all but the last five decades – often means the nutrients in the soil are provided externally, i.e. from a sack of fertilisers, leaving the soil increasingly denuded. Farming organically is good for soil health and without healthy soil we're all stuffed. This was one good thing we learned all those years ago on The Black Isle when we were hippies. Organically growing was obscure and largely unheard of back then but the reasons behind it remain as cogent and apt then as now.

Call me a sensitive wuss if you must but I don't want to eat more pesticide or herbicide residue than I have to and that gunk is on there, trust me. PAN UK, an organisation which used to be known as the Pesticide Trust, cites studies that have shown the following:

> Ninety-three per cent of non-organic oranges analysed contained pesticide residues, 78 per cent of apples analysed contained pesticide residues, 43 per cent of all fruit and vegetables analysed had detectable levels of pesticides, 50 per cent of lettuce contained residues from seven or more chemicals, 71 per cent of cereal bars with pesticide residues, 83 per cent of oily fish showed pesticide residues.

All of this may only be small amounts each time but those small amounts add up to a uniquely blended cocktail of toxins inside of you and it's not a good cocktail. It's not exactly a Long Island Iced Tea, in fact it's probably nearer to Agent Orange. The consequences of this constant, day after day, week after week, year after year consumption is unknown and hard to test. It may have a lot, some or no effect on us. There is no way to know for sure. I don't think it's being overly paranoid to be concerned with such issues. But it doesn't just stop there. Organic farming standards have lots of other implications in terms of welfare and environment.

The Soil Association, which is the hand-spun jumper-wearing head honcho of the organic movement in the UK, tell us,

> Artificial chemical fertilisers are prohibited – instead organic farmers develop a healthy, fertile soil by growing and rotating a mixture of crops, adding organic matter such as compost or manure and using clover to fix nitrogen from the atmosphere. Pesticides are severely restricted – instead organic farmers develop nutrient-rich soil to grow strong,

healthy crops and encourage wildlife to help control pests and disease.

But it doesn't stop there, animal welfare is at the heart of the system and a truly free-range life for farm animals is guaranteed. Also a diversity of crops and animals are raised on the farm and rotated over several seasons, including fallow periods. This mixed farming approach helps break cycles of pests and disease and builds fertility in the soil. The routine use of drugs, antibiotics and wormers is banned – instead the farmer will use preventative methods, like moving animals to fresh pasture and keeping smaller herd and flock sizes.

This is much nearer to how animals and crops have been farmed for centuries before the knee-jerk use of artificial fertilisers, herbicides and pesticides to maximise production. It looks after the fertility of the soil in order to grow wholesome vegetables and fruit, and provides meat which is more likely to be stress and toxin free. What's not to like about that?

If you're a vegetarian or vegan, remember most organic vegetables are grown using manure from farmed animals which means if you don't want to exploit animals you cannot eat it and must source food that has been grown using non-animal fertilisers such as seaweed. They do exist. We used to use seaweed we'd picked ourselves in our garden on the Black Isle back in 1983. How far ahead of our time where we? Goddamn freaks.

But while I know it's not perfect I think it's about as good as we're going to get when food needs to be grown en masse. There are always going to be times when you can't get an organic option, which is another reason why you should always get organic when you can because you are almost certainly going to have to take on board some non-organic toxins on a regular basis anyway – so why add to them? Naturally, if you wake up one morning and have grown a second head and can't afford to feed another mouth, you might want to make your diet 100 per cent organic.

Buying organic doesn't mean you have to be a middle-class woman called Sophie or a New-Age hippy type. It's marketed to those people but if you're not one of them, it should not exclude you. All we want is pure, unadulterated food. 'Give me spots on the apples and give me the birds and the bees,' as Joni Mitchell sang in 'Big Yellow Taxi' forty years ago. It's not really changed, except that DDT, an insecticide sung about in that song (possibly the only insecticide ever mentioned in the pantheon of rock 'n' roll), is now illegal because it turns out though it's great at killing bugs, it has the potential to mimic hormones and thereby disrupt endocrine systems in wildlife and possibly humans. Call me old fashioned but I like my endocrine system undisrupted.

Obviously, if you can grow your own food, or even just some of it, so much the better. When we moved from Edinburgh to Norfolk, we took over a large garden where we set about growing all the stuff it's hard to buy organically grown from supermarkets, such as black cabbage, fennel, purple sprouting broccoli and globe artichoke. All incredibly middle-class foods, I know, though quite why, I have no idea. Why are some fruit and vegetables middle-class in this country when others are not? What dictates it? Alas the intricacies of the British class system are beyond the scope of this book.

So to sum up, organic is better for you. The way it is grown is better for the soil. It is better for the animals you are ultimately going to feast on so you owe it to yourself to eat it wherever and whenever you can – even if the uncool people think you're mad. One further good thing about choosing organic: there's much less choice and thus makes life much more simple. I consider this a huge advantage!

FREE RANGE

While I've now accepted that eating animals isn't morally objectionable, even if you don't kill them yourself there's no reason to give them a hard time. Keeping them in surroundings where they can thrive and live comfortable, stress-free lives seems a decent trade off against whacking them and feasting on their flesh and organs dontcha think? Not least because it produces better, more nutritious, healthier, tastier, more tender meat.

Intensive factory farming of animals is good for profits and for production of cheap food and that's enough for some people. They're just animals, after all, they would say. Then again, so are we. But just because we can do that to animals is no reason why we should, is it? It doesn't make any sense as a consumer because it doesn't produce as good a quality food. Remember, intensively farmed animals are fed soya-based, high-protein feeds and wheat to make them grow super quick and that affects the nutritional composition of the meat.

So I look for free-range meat and eggs and would never buy anything that was produced intensively. Don't be fooled by words like Farm Fresh. It just means it comes from a massive unit in conditions that would make the apocalypse look like a day in paradise. If it doesn't say it's free range, it means it isn't. Organic meat and eggs are always free range.

BEEF

When it comes to beef, all cows are just fed on grass aren't they? No they're not. Though that's what you'd think isn't it? Cow in field. It's a common enough sight. Most, though not all, are at some point also fed wheat and soya meal as a high-protein feed which, as previously mentioned negatively affects the omega-3 and omega-6 balance. And also, let's be honest, it's just not natural for a bovine animal to eat soya or wheat, so how likely is it that it will produce natural and healthy animals that will feed us well? Not as likely as feeding them on what they're designed to eat, I'd argue. To me, that just sounds sensible. I also only buy British beef because it seems mad to pay money to fly it in when so much is grown here.

CHICKEN AND DUCK

Chickens are designed to scratch in and around woodland. They should get a varied diet that way. But intensively reared birds are fed on wheat and soya to make them grow quickly and if they're kept for eggs, layers pellets too. By and large the same thing goes for ducks. It's like fast food for them and unnatural by any definition. You might as well send them out to McDonalds to eat and then make them sit on the sofa all day. Most would say it means the birds have more flavour when kept as a woodland creature and are living like they should, not in some massive shed growing as fast as possible. If you buy organic, too, it means that you're not eating birds that have been given growth promoters or antibiotics. It also keeps the omega-3 and -6 balance at their natural levels in the meat. This means you're being fed properly. Remember, This is a Good Thing!

PORK

Pigs that are left to snort around in the mud and forage for food the way their ancestors, wild boars, did means you're getting a slow-grown porker, which means great flavour and a happy pig – happy at least until the moment it gets a bolt through its head. Sorry piggy, it's a human-eat-animal world, you'd do the same thing to us if you could. Because your natural pigmeister is a fatty creature, it's especially important to eat them organically grown. Toxins from pesticides and anything else they acquire from feed or environment is stored readily in their fat. So you'll consume more of it if you feast on the crackling.

LAMB

Lambs are killed young, obviously, so tend not to be fed on much high-protein meal but are still a fatty animal, which is again a good argument for only eating organic. We should be eating British lamb and not New Zealand. You don't have to be a flag-waving, jingoistic, Union Jack waistcoat wearing patriot to think that. It's just mental to fly corpses of lambs half way around the world. Who thinks it makes any sense when there's plenty of lamb here? Even if there was no lamb here, it's still wacko to spend all that energy to get it here from 10,000 miles away.

VENISON

Go for wild not farmed if you can get it: it will have lived off all manner of vegetation and won't have had any or much in the way of additional feeding if it's been roaming through the Glens playing the bagpipes and wearing the full kilt.

Chinese Water Deer and Monk Jack live all around our place in Norfolk; they wander through the garden and eat everything given the slightest chance. Cute little things they are too, looking more like a small kangaroo than a deer. They're good eating, though wild Scottish venison is a more powerful, rich-tasting beastie. Whichever you get, make sure you cook it with lots of fat because it's very lean and therefore can be quite dry.

GAME

Whether it's rabbit, quail, pheasant or anything else, if you can get a caught or shot wild animal then so much the better. If Ted Nugent is your neighbour this should be no problem but unless you've seen a long-haired man with disconcertingly wild eyes firing a lot of semi-automatic weaponry in the back garden, he probably isn't. Commercially produced pheasant are fed on wheat routinely. Booo. Go for really wild game if you can get it.

BACON

I buy bacon that isn't made with sodium nitrate. Some reckon too much nitrate is carcinogenic. Not instantly, of course. You don't eat a slice and that's it. It's a long-term thing. But you can end up eating nitrate regularly if you enjoy preserved meats, bacon and sausages a lot so it is something to be aware of. I do occasionally buy organic nitrated bacon figuring, hell, a dose of nitrate now and again won't kill me. I might be wrong but Death by Bacon is a good way to go, I reckon. You won't get non-nitrate bacon on the High Street or in your supermarket; it's too non-conventional for twenty-first-century food purveyors. This is where the internet is your friend. Order it through the mail and it arrives in an envelope. Bacon en papillote. Lovely. I get ours from Laverstoke Park.

NUTS AND SEEDS

Avoid peanuts because they're full of carbs and too easy to eat a large bucket of once you get sat in front of the TV. Everything else is fine but don't eat your body weight in them as they do contain some carbs and at some point eating a lot of calorie-dense food will put lard on your arse. Obviously go for organic. I eat brazils, cashews, pumpkins seeds and macadamia nuts most, with a few pecans thrown in occasionally. If they've grown in a hard shell it often protects them more from any pesticides so don't panic if you can't get organic versions of them. Keep them in the freezer, not the fridge – like all those bottles of vegetable oil, they're full of polyunsaturated fat so they're not stable and go rancid very easily. Freezing keeps them fresh. It's surprisingly nice eating a chilled nut. Macadamias are more like a savoury hard ice cream, which you may never have even dreamed about but I assure you is very satisfying.

GELATINE

This is great stuff and under-rated as a food. You buy it in sheets, soften it and stir it into fruit or milk jellies. Gelatine is made from the collagen in bones, trotters, hooves or any other stuff on an animal that can be boiled up. It's virtually all protein and is good for your joints. No, sheesh, not for *those* sort of joints. You can't smoke it. You could try but I'm betting it gives you a headache, like banana skins and morning glory seeds.

MILK & DAIRY

Choose raw, organic and unhomegenised milk over pasteurised, homogenised stuff if you can.

When I was young, unpasteurised 'green-top' milk was commonplace. However, it dropped out of fashion as pasteurisation supposedly guaranteed milk free from bacterial contamination, especially from TB which used to be of great concern. By the mid 1970s pasteurised milk completely dominated the market but it was still often not homogenised. I know our daily pints of milk from the milk man – how quaint the idea of milk man sounds now – were not homogenised because we always had to shake the bottle to disperse the cream on the top of the bottle.

We eventually bought raw Jersey milk direct from a farm in Herefordshire called John's Jersey's which arrived mail order.

As soon as I poured it, it was obviously a different product all together. For a start it was more creamy yellow in colour from all that lovely fat. And the taste … man oh man it took me right back to childhood and the days of green-top milk.

It has a more buttermilk quality to it; it feels smooth and silky in the mouth. It is wholly different to any milk you will have tasted unless you were born around forty or fifty years ago. It is how milk used to be in a time when there was almost no lactose intolerance. When you taste pasteurised milk afterwards it has a 'cooked' taste to it, still nice enough but not as fresh in flavour. The cream from raw milk is also stunning; thick, almost solid and with a rich, almost caramel flavour to it.

Today almost all milk is homogenised, which people tell me is achieved by squirting it through a fine sieve against a hard surface to smash up the fat molecules. Great, eh? Just so you don't have to shake a bottle. Have we gone certifiably insane? Yes people, we've invented a process to distribute fat through milk evenly when we used to just shake the bloody bottle. Talk about bleedin' bourgeois. How fat and lazy have we become that we're too weak and indolent to shake our own milk? Did we ask for this to happen? What sort of freak asks for milk to be pre-shook up?

Some researchers believe that these battered and bruised modified fat molecules are deleterious to our health. It's been messed around with for no good reason at all. It also increases the price of the milk because it is a process which has to be paid for. Do you really want this state of affairs?

Not that the dairy industry is bothered. All of this allows a mass-produced, mass-market, samey product. And to be fair, people seem to like it like that. People have been convinced to buy semi-skimmed and skimmed milk for fear of having a big fat greasy heart attack and so that is where the high demand is these days. By skimming out the fat, you are of course losing most of what is best about milk, leaving a watery excuse behind with much less nutrition but hey, we're so freakin' wealthy we can do what we like. See how rich we are, we can take the best shit out of food and throw it away. Yeehaw!

Yeah and you know what's happened since this has become the way to present milk for sale, don't you? The rise and rise of lactose intolerance, that's what. Rare when I was a kid, it's now commonplace. This hasn't happened for no reason. It isn't a plague from the Great Cow God Moo. Those who care about such matters relate this to the pasteurisation and homogenisation of milk. We are messing with something basic and natural; something honest and straight forward has been warped into a mass-produced industrial fluid.

But when it comes to milk, the woo-woo-my-head-is-on-fire madness does not stop there. The really healthy, nutritious raw milk, the unadulterated, as we've always drank it for millennia milk, is virtually illegal! Yes, illegal! The laws in England and Wales restrict its sale to the farm gate or via mail order. They can't sell it into stores. In Scotland it is even more crazy. It is 100 per cent illegal to sell it even from your own farm. Yeah, I mean the Scots don't need something nutritious or healthy to drink do they? No, they've only got the worst health record in Europe, why would they need something that feeds them well? Well, call the cops if you want but we bought raw milk mail order and had it sent to our apartment in Scotland. So bust me. Do the Lothian and

Borders police have a special Milk Squad to bust anyone who brings in milk that has not been pre-heated? It is a bloody stupid law.

If you can't get raw milk, buy organic unpasteurised or just organic pasteurised if they've taken your freedom to buy that away as well.

If you can buy hard cheese made from raw milk, and it's not exactly commonplace, then so much the better. If not, your first option should be organic unpasteurised soft cheeses and then organic hard cheeses. Goat's cheese is rarely produced on an industrial scale and can be a good option too.

Needless to say, if you have a local cheese shop this is where you should be heading and not to your local enormo-dome of food conformity.

I never saw the attraction of cream until I bought some raw rich double Jersey Cream from John's Jerseys, a farm in Wales. It's extra double-thick raw cream and is astonishing stuff, full of rich buttery flavour. If you can't get raw, go for any organic cream. I eat some cream most days. Not a tanker full of it but some. It hasn't put any fat on me. I don't expect it will either not even when a doctor frowns and adopts a patronising tone and talks to me like I'm nine years old.

FATS

When it comes to cooking fats, use only lard, duck or goose fat and extra virgin coconut oil. They don't deteriorate at high heats. Use butter if you're not heating it too much. Organic olive oil is also good for salads etc. Don't cook with it as it denudes with heat.

Don't be afraid to eat slices of butter as though it's cheese, similarly a spoonful of coconut oil is delicious – it melts in the mouth. There are coconut evangelicals who swear by it as a panacea for all manner of modern illnesses. Some say it actually makes you lose weight. I adore it and even use it as a moisturiser, OK, OK, you can stop laughing now. Try it and then we'll see who's crazy. It works better than Oil of Olay for a fraction of the price, aye, because I'm worth it. Whatever you use, stop worrying about good quality fat. It's food not poison.

FRUIT AND VEGETABLES

I avoid anything with a high-carb content so potatoes are off limits unless I'm physically very active all the time and need them to fuel me. Yeah everyone else eats them but hell, you've met the public haven't you? And you want to be like them? Do me a favour. I don't bother with sweet potatoes much either but apart from that you can feast on pretty much whatever you like. If it fits in your mouth, try it. This is my advice for the bedroom and the kitchen.

While you want to be buying organic, chances are you won't always be able to. In that case I always avoid non-organic leaves because they'll have been subject to the full chemical spray, whereas self-covering veg like savoy cabbages are safer once you strip off the outside leaves. Don't buy non organic lettuce as it's one of the most pesticide-drenched of all. Similarly soft skin fruits like strawberries have probably been sprayed most so go for harder things like apples or pears if you're not getting organic.

See what a hell of a dance we have to go through just to get food to eat that might not poison us? Honestly, if you came to earth from another universe, you'd think this was the Bizarro World. 'Why are you putting poisons on the stuff that is supposed to keep your species alive?' Christ knows Space Boy and you can put that probe down too if you don't mind.

Don't try and fill up on veg though, use fat to satiate your appetite. I tend to major on berries because they're low in sugar; I don't eat bananas because they're too sweet and starchy. If you don't have berries go for apples and pears but, as each one has around twenty grams of carbohydrates, you only need a couple each day at the most. Avoid any very sugary fruit such as melon.

Stay away from fruit juice. I've actually now stopped drinking it because it suddenly struck me as a bizarre intense form of freaky food. A kind of processed food in fact.

Squeeze an orange and see how much juice you get out of it – it's not much, A standard 250ml glass is like eating seven or eight oranges. You'd never do that. You'd never eat more than two at one time because the fibre from the orange would fill you up. Your body naturally regulates consumption in that way but by drinking fruit juice, you're by-passing that regulation.

It comes in a big carton so we pour it out by the glassful thinking that it's healthy, so drinking more has to be more healthy. Wrong. It's a bit mad really. We expect our digestive system to handle anything we throw at it in any quantity. It must piss our guts right off. 'What the hell are they doing throwing all this sugary stuff down us? Right, everybody out. We're going on strike.' I used to get rotten indigestion from fruit juice and acid reflux when I was a big fat lad. Fruit juice is a big hit of fructose which spikes your insulin and may contribute to weight gain. I know it sounds weird saying fat doesn't make you fat and fruit juice does – but it's true. My gran would have nodded sagely, pulled on a fag and said bitterly, 'I could have told you that for nothing, daft lad.'

FISH

For me, farmed fish isn't really very cool at all. It sounds OK doesn't it? A big loch somewhere in Scotland full of salmon.

It sounds fairly natural really but ha, it bloody isn't. Farmed fish are often a poor imitation of wild fish. It's almost certainly been fed on soya and high-protein meal and as a result is much higher in omega-6. And if that still doesn't sound bad enough, read this from The Fish Site:

> Farmed salmon are fed meal and oils from wild-caught fish. Each pound of salmon produced requires at least three pounds of wild-caught fish, challenging the presumption that fish farming necessarily reduces commercial fishing pressure. In fact, there is a net loss of protein in the marine ecosystem as a whole when wild catch is converted into meal for aquaculture consumption.

Hello again Bizarro World. We're feeding wild fish to farmed fish! Do you want that done for you, really? Doesn't it seem ... err ... fucking insane? Why not eat the wild fish instead?

Of course, the fish may well be dyed if it's salmon because they believe the idiot public like their fish to be brightly coloured. Maybe they do. That's no excuse. Plenty of environmentalistas also object to how fish farms pollute their habitat with a lot of fish pooh. As they're intensively farmed they get all sorts of infestations which then escape into the rivers and streams and infect the wild salmon who are. understandably enough, very pissed off about this turn of events. Not quite pissed enough not to breed with escaped salmon though, thus diluting the pure wild fish stock further. No matter how natural and bucolic it looks on the packet, if it doesn't say it's wild, it's farmed and that is a whole world of crazy hurt.

Watch out for smoked fish that hasn't been smoked but flavoured or dyed yellow. Some think you should restrict how much smoked foods you eat, fearing it will be carcinogenic if you eat it too much. Others think it's just overly paranoid and there are worse things than a bit of naturally smoked fish to worry about. I'm inclined to agree. Then again, I've only just discovered the wonders of the Craster kipper. Also, smoking fish was a common thing long before the prevalence of degenerative diseases so if it is cancer inducing it seems likely to be so because of its relationship with something else in the modern diet. Irn Bru, possibly.

The occasional tin of salmon is a useful thing to have in stock – make sure it's also wild, furious even. Tinned salmon was a great favourite of my grandparents but it was only, and I really do mean only, ever for tea on a Sunday. Why it was reserved for this almost holy status I'm not sure, but it was always there, served with a stick of celery, an eye-wateringly strong spring onion, slices of tomato, radishes and cucumber. This was a salad. Nothing else qualified for eating raw and thus could not be called a salad. They were hardline about such things. It was adorned with one of their few processed foods, Heinz Salad Cream. A great treat – one dollop only though, two was pure hedonism.

We eat a lot of frozen fish because it's more convenient though not as good as fresh fish. Coley is always cheap and is superior to cod in my view. I wish there were more frozen white fish in the supermarkets than just cod and haddock and plaice. I don't know how it's ended up being the trio and little else when there are so many others swimming around our seas. We seem trapped in a 'no one buys it so no one fishes-it-so no one buys it' circle. We're mad. The seas are loaded with all sorts of fish; like Gran said, 'get it bloody eaten'.

DRINKS

Perhaps I'm weird but the fact that every person on earth seems to drink cans of fizzy pop really does my head in – as you may have guessed in the previous chapter. All that sugar, all those artificial sweeteners and fuck-with-your-brain flavourings. I mean, just how did it become so cool, so bloody requisite to have your hand wrapped around one of these cans every day, several times a day? Is it the colour of the cans, the logos, the taste or all of the above? Maybe they're really properly addictive. Maybe they're compulsive like crack cocaine.

Here's a really far out idea, if you want to quench your thirst … drink water! If you want a buzz, take a hit of some liquor or if you want something liquid and nutritional choose milk. If you really want a headache, bang your head against a wall instead, it will probably do you less damage than all those artificial sweeteners.

I'm not trying to be holier-than-thou, honestly, even though this will sound like any pretentious sod you'll ever meet, but green tea is actually my beverage of choice. My gran would have hated green tea. She thought all tea should be dark orange and strong enough to stand a teaspoon up in. She thought drinking tea black was akin to devil worship, though she frowned upon sugar in tea as some sort of moral weakness. 'Have you seen how much sugar he puts in his tea?' she would say, if she wanted to suggest someone was not quite trustworthy.

Green tea is another poncy middle-class comestible though isn't it? Again, I don't know why. It hasn't made me middle class. Not so's you'd notice anyway. I've not started wearing linen suits or going to the opera, nor have I learned how to make small talk without offending anyone, which, to me, seems to be an art form the proper middle class have mastered. Drinking green tea hasn't elevated me onto a higher spiritual plain, though occasionally adverts for the stuff suggest it might well do.

There is much written about how good for you green tea polyphenols are. These are a type of antioxidant which zooms around your body hoovering up nasty stuff. See, I know all the medical terms. Did you know that green tea contains salubrious polyphenolsand catechins, the most abundant of which is epigallocatechin gallate. Whoo hoo! I love a bit of epigallocatechin gallate. Well who doesn't? Weren't they a prog rock band in the 1970s?

Green tea is one of those things for which a new health claim seems to appear every week. There is nothing it can't help with, from macular degeneration to cancer to weight loss. I'm sure if you made trousers out of green tea leaves someone would claim it makes your legs go faster. I like green tea and I do think it's good for me, but I don't think it can be quite as good for me as the dozens of health claims suggest it is. However, compared to Pepsi or Coke it is the elixir of life.

I'll also drink pretty much any pure herbal tea, especially peppermint and camomile. Watch out for those with 'natural flavourings' in. They're often in the ones which look most natural such as Good Earth Lemongrass Green Tea. We don't know what those flavourings are and they won't tell us so, sorry fella, that's a no sale. Trust no one.

I don't drink coffee though plenty of people do. Since changing my diet I've felt little need for the energy boost coffee gives you when you're flagging so it's another one of those things I've dumped. Some say it's good for you in many and varied ways, helping everything from liver function to gout. Mind you others say it'll give you cancer and heart disease. I bet it doesn't. Not right away, anyway. There'd be corpses littered all over branches of Starbucks if it did and that would be bad for business

Like many people, I don't do well on too much caffeine.

It gives me palpitations and headaches and I reckon that's not a good enough trade off for the taste of coffee. I once had coffee at Betty's Tea Shop in Harrogate that was so strong I swear I began to hallucinate. I began to think it was actually the 1930s and I was surrounded by a hundred Miss Marples dressed in tweed twin sets. Someone must have put dope in the Fat Rascals.

Some people swear by coffee enemas and possibly swear while having coffee enemas. Why? Is it simple perversion to put coffee up your arse? Well, possibly. But it is also supposed to be a very good way to detox your colon. If you feel your colon needs detoxing. How do you know if it does? Is there a dial on your arse that tells you? I've never done it, I hasten to add. I'm too squeamish about such matters, but Dawn has done it a few times and says it's rather good fun. Well it's something to do on the long dark nights out here in the deepest rural Norfolk.

I stay away from beer and lager as they're high in carbs. I know it seems like life will end but it won't and you'll feel bloody great once you quit them. Get a refund for a faulty life off God if you don't.

Your choice for booze is white spirits such as vodka, gin or lovely, lovely brush cleaner. Failing that dry white wine is a good old standby. Don't use mixers such as tonic water as it's loaded with artificial sweeteners and quinine which is really only good if your heart has stopped and you need it to be jolted back into life in which case you won't feel much like drinking.

Instead use plain fizzy water with your gin. It's a brilliant drink, much cleaner and sophisticated in flavour and 100 per cent natural. Bartenders think you're very strange but everyone. and I do mean everyone, who tries it, prefers it over the traditional gin and tonic eventually. It really is a much cooler drink.

VEGETABLE OIL

The more I read, the more I feel vegetable oils are at the heart of so many health and weight issues. They're so unnatural, so industrially produced, so high in omega-6 and I'm not convinced that our bodies have any idea what to do with them, especially once they've been subjected to heat which damages them and turns them into free radicals.

You think I'm weird? Well I'm not the one who has set up massive industrial oil extraction plants to strip oil out of soy beans or corn cobs when perfectly good, healthy, easily obtained alternatives are available.

Worse yet, most vegetable oils are horrible. What would you rather eat, a spoon of butter or a spoon of corn oil? Polyunsaturated oils are not stable, they go rancid and then essentially poison us. Free radicals, which admittedly does sound like a name that should have been given to a hippy commune somewhere out in Marin County, California, well they mess your body up. Think about it this way, if the oil has to be extracted by an industrial process, then it's already so processed that you shouldn't really want to eat it when better unprocessed natural alternatives exist like lard or duck fat or butter which have been used for centuries, long before anyone worried about saturated fat killing them.

The only oil in our house is olive oil. Squeeze an olive and the deal is done. You don't have to process it, bleach it, filter it or stroke it nicely and call it darling. It is what it is, you eat it or you don't. Easy. As these things should be. Why should they be any more difficult, complex or industrial? Do we think we're being clever? We're not. It's idiocy.

GRAINS

Another easy one this: I don't eat any. Well not unless you count wild rice which is a grass and not a grain at all apparently. Who knew? It looks and tastes like you're eating grass though. This might sound as attractive as eating earwigs but it's really good eating. Sort of smoky and chewy. I have a little wild rice a couple of times a week. Maybe three spoonfuls. Yeah, I know, I'm living like a crazy man. If you need a bit of flour to thicken a gravy or to coat a piece of fish, I use a dusting of tapioca. I also use brown rice breadcrumbs to make a batter for fish with. It's not exactly living high on the hog but whatever gets you through the night, I say.

I just don't eat any wheat. Not ever. Why not? Because it is grown by evil pixies hell bent on making us sick, that's why. No, not really. Well sort of. Look, we can eat wheat, it'll go in our mouths and we can swallow it. As animals we've been eating it for quite a long time, perhaps as long as 10,000 years but not nearly as long as we have not been eating it.

But, as I talked about earlier, the kind of grain we used to eat back then is not the kind of grain available now. Nothing like it. It's changed radically as it's been hybridised, especially in the last couple of decades.

Even if it wasn't screwing up our digestive systems, it is really easy to over-eat wheat because you only ever eat it in a cooked and processed format as pie crusts, biscuits, cakes or bread. All of which can be quickly eaten in large amounts before it makes you feel full.

Wheat sounds natural but it really isn't. It's a highly contrived crop which we're familiar with so we think it's as natural as the trees and the sky. It's not actually that high in nutrition either. Don't forget that most industrially produced bread is made with fortified flour precisely because there isn't much in the way of nutrition in wheat. So it's not as if, by excluding it from your diet, you're missing out on something you can't get elsewhere.

If you eat wholewheat flour, good luck with the

indigestion. I ate it for years, hell, I even ground my own in a big hand-turned mill at one point (you've got to love a hippy's dedication to living like its 1734). It's certainly full of impossible-to-digest, insoluble fibre which you will pass out but, look, that's not the only way you can keep your poop chute well-oiled. If you eat fruit and vegetables you get fibre which is much less harsh on your digestive system and will stop you from becoming what my gran used to call 'egg bound', though as far as I know she never actually laid any eggs.

My life has immeasurably improved since I quit eating wheat, maybe others don't suffer as much, perhaps some suffer more – all colours in the spectrum seem likely. I have tried bread three times since quitting it. Each time it gave me indigestion and a vaguely sore feeling in my guts, though this may well have been a loopy, psychosomatic response as I sat there, trying to listen to what my body was saying, though it was probably actually saying, 'Why the hell are you sitting there waiting for me to say something, I'm your body, I don't talk, remember?'

You won't miss eating wheat, trust me, I'm not a doctor. What you might miss is the things that are used to flavour wheat. You might miss pizza but how often did you just eat a pizza base with nothing on? You might miss toast but you never ate it dry. You might miss biscuits but they're always sweetened and flavoured. In other words, it's the flavourings that you're missing not the wheat itself, most of the time. So just keep eating tasty food and as long as you do so, life goes on as normal. It's not a big deal.

To sceptics I'd say, just try not eating wheat for a couple of weeks because nothing bad will happen to you. You won't hallucinate, you won't end up in the foetal position weeping, you won't shake uncontrollably. Just see how you feel. If you don't like it, then open up and swallow some wheat again.

It's easy. If you don't try it, you'll never know what it's like. And you'll never know how it might make you feel. Secretly, you know it's actually quite a cool thing to do if only because everyone stands in line and eats wheat like a massive herd of cattle, endlessly feeding on it, getting bigger and bigger and bigger, thoughtlessly shovelling it in. Why not break the cycle and be different?

BEANS AND PULSES

I lived off them for twenty-six years though I never felt comfortable with the word pulses. It sounds like you're eating a heartbeat. They're rich in carbs and often hard to digest but I'm not suggesting an occasional spoon of Puy lentils will destroy your health – that would be bonkers. For years I thought they were good protein but it turns out they're really not as they're lacking in a few of the essential amino acids. They are however ideal if you are going in for a fart-lighting contest. For decades, the only beans anyone ate were baked beans but now exhortations to eat them are commonplace from the healthy eating lobby, who are wedded to the idea that some form of protein that doesn't contain saturated fat is always superior for your health.

SWEETENERS

This one is easy, I don't use any. Not honey, not agave, not maple syrup. Just because they're in your local health food shop and hippies think they're better and more hip than sugar, doesn't mean anything. It's all pure carbohydrate.

And that's your food sorted. Easy. Less choice plus better quality equals more happiness. It's generally the way to go. Now, as you may have noticed, I'm not your typical wassock who might write a book about food or a loopy diet. I know all of this sounds like a massive departure from what you and I know as 'normal' eating. And let's not pretend that it isn't. It damn well is. It's freaky weird, man. But there's nothing wrong with freaky weird. Without freaky weird there'd never be any progress. When Sir Isaac Newton came up with all those ideas about gravity after the business with the apple, someone somewhere would have been saying, 'That Newton dude, he's whacked out. He's always messing with the apples in my orchard. I'm going to kick his ass.'

But let's escape the here and now for a moment and travel back in time. If you don't have a time machine, or good quality psychotropic drugs, then use your imagination. One hundred and fifty years ago, a life without processed food would be entirely normal for your working-class Joe. A life without much or any sugar would also be quite typical. Go back 350 years and you wouldn't be eating that much wheat, just some rough wholegrain bread and maybe some oat groats. You wouldn't be eating any potatoes either as they were fancy and modern and mistrusted until well into the eighteenth century. Your grains would be pretty unsophisticated, spelt-types. Go back another few thousand years and here we are as hunter-gatherers, a-huntin' 'n' a gatherin'. They call me the wanderer, I wander round and round and round and round. All of that vibe. Life is brutal and Waitrose don't deliver.

What's this time travel all about? Just that now is not forever. Yes now is all we have in life and is so powerful an experience that it feels as though it has lasted and will last forever. It seems to be all there is and all there can ever be and all there ever was. But in reality, what we think of as everyday and normal and familiar is actually just the latest phase or trend. My ancestors who lived in the east Yorkshire countryside 150 years ago would recognise and understand my diet today, much more than they would have recognised it when I was a vegetarian.

What I'm saying is, don't be afraid of the new just because it seems different. It is actually the modern, supermarket-centric diet that is weird and out of whack; the departure from history and tradition. The aisle and aisles of manu-factured products would seem incredible to our ancestors. Even when I was a kid it was inconceivable that so much food would be available under one roof; that so many products would be vying for our attention and money.

While the twenty-first century supermarket has its use and its attractions, I believe it is corrupting us from the inside out. Not just in terms of nutrition but because all our food experiences have now been homogenised by the super-market experience. When you pull all your food out of a big warehouse once a week and everything is always available, there are no individual unique stories to tell people about say, the first strawberries of the season that your mam or granddad brought home from your local green grocer. It's all been subsumed in the mass corporate experience of 365-days a year, twenty-four hours, seven days a week, everything all the time. The Sainstrosetescoification of life.

This is not a good thing because it smoothes out life's individual textures and stories. It might make life easier but it makes it less interesting.

I've emerged from this adventure being totally against all forms of processed food. By eating them you are handing over the control of what keeps you alive to someone else. It's up to them what they put in it, you just have to swallow it. Cook everything from scratch and you have the power. You rule and you get the benefits both nutritional and also psychological. You have seized the reins of your own life and are controlling the show instead of being controlled. You are the puppet master not the puppet. It's about freedom and independence and not being a lab rat for the food processing industry whose interest is in their profit and not your health. Remember, it's not their job to make healthy food for you, it's their job to make profitable food for themselves – the rest of it is just marketing bullshit.

If it means you've got to spend more on food – though it doesn't always – then that's what you have to do.

In the 1970s we used to spend on average 25 per cent of our budget on food, now it's around 11 or 12 per cent. Yes we all want to spend more of our money on new electronics, expensive shirts or holidays on hot beaches. But if the choice is between these things and hitting yourself in the face with a brick, which in health terms it is – and worse – then what's your choice going to be? C'mon, you know what's right.

The trend in the twenty-first century is to say that everything is shit. That everything has got worse and is more expensive. Someone even wrote a book called *Is it Just Me or is Everything Shit?* It was him. There's never been a golden age, life has always been a veil of freakin' tears, especially for the poor and the down-trodden. But although no one likes or wants to admit or appreciate the fact, food really has got much cheaper in real terms over the last three decades.

But this is not a good thing if it makes you sick, perform poorly and die young unless this trio of miseries is what turns your love light on. Surely the point of this being upright on two legs and wandering around gig, is to have a bloody good time and to enjoy the physicality of existence, not drag your fat arse around, sweating like a pig in a jumper and feeling like dirt just because you ate the wrong food for years. It makes no sense to do that now, does it? It's what I did for too damn long.

Someone said to me that they loved beer, chips and pies so

much that the quality of their life would be seriously diminished if they adopted a diet that excluded those things. It's understandable as a viewpoint. At least it would be if it was genuinely true. But I don't think it really is. Such beliefs are delusions and habituations.

Yes it is a wonderfully satisfying triumvirate of foods and if you are wedded to the notion that your quality of life is dictated by eating them, I doubt there is much point in arguing otherwise. Might as well not even waste time thinking about it. Get on with your life. Nothing to see here.

If you are hard wired into these food choices and do not want to do without them, then fine, it's your choice and who am I or anyone else to tell you it's wrong. If you're eating them and you feel great then maybe there's no reason to stop, not yet anyway. You might be run over tomorrow; life can quickly evaporate. If Sting has taught us anything, and on balance that doesn't seem likely, it's how fragile we are.

That being said, I know for a fact that many people feel their health in all sorts of different ways is not as good as it could be, that their quality of life is poorer than they'd like it to be, that what they eat plays a big part in that, perhaps the biggest part. If that's the case and giving up chips, pies and beer makes you feel a lot better, makes you happier and healthier, I suspect it will seem little hardship to give them up. It's a trade-off well worth it.

I loved all three as much as anyone but never pay the fact that I don't eat them anymore a second thought. I have no wish to eat them any more than I have a wish to eat my own underwear. This makes me think that such things, though they seem to give our lives much added pleasure, is really something of an illusion. It is just the pleasure of eating tasty food we crave and enjoy. As long as you continue to do that, you don't feel like you're missing out or being deprived in any way. So you might think you love pies, chips and beer, but what you really love is tasty food.

Besides, the reality of life is far less black and white. We don't *always* love the foods and drinks that we think we love. In other words, sometimes we eat them and it doesn't quite do the job. There are times when a cold beer feels like nectar from the gods and others, probably the majority of the time in fact, when it's just something you drink out of habit and it doesn't deliver the same peak of satisfaction. It is the peak we recall when we think of doing without it, not the more mundane, habitual consumption experiences.

Same goes for so many foods we hold dear in our personal pleasure domes. Habits are hard to break, so hard that they turn into unshakable beliefs. This is why you end up thinking, God, I can't live without chips, they're so brilliant, forgetting all the soggy, limp chips you've had in your life. It might seem unimaginable to do without them but this is all a delusion.

And something else needs to be said and I know my gran would approve of this. When it comes to food, we can't just have what we want when we want it. Or rather, we can, but we shouldn't think this is either a good thing or indeed something we should judge the quality of our lives by.

Just because we have massive supermarkets full of tens of thousands of foodstuffs doesn't mean we have to eat all of them. Choosing not to eat something that will certainly fit in your mouth and might taste nice but which will, in the short or long term, make you less healthy, is not the same thing as deprivation. Not having what you want all the time is not the same thing as deprivation, either. We shouldn't behave like spoiled brats.

Making the right food choices for you and your well-being might mean exercising some discipline in the widest sense, but that is something to appreciate, not to feel depressed about. Perhaps we've been sold an idea that we can have it all; if we can afford it it's ours and that this self-indulgence is the marker for the quality and success of your life. This in itself causes over-eating as we seek to gorge ourselves to prove our own success.

But the best lived lives are not those with the most stuff bought or eaten. In fact the prosperity of our health relies on us not doing that. We need to refocus our minds to understand that.

...AND IN THE END

After spending eighteen months looking into what happened to me, reorganising my brain, re-shaping my life, ditching twenty-six years of assumption and ignorance and uncovering this world of lower-carb, higher natural fats and protein eating, I'm left feeling a bit puzzled.

It's self-evident that the information status quo on healthy eating is delivering worse and worse results and we've seen that much of the reasoning behind it is either severely flawed or certainly questionable.

So why is the healthy eating advice still so hard line? Why doesn't it change?

I'm not prone to conspiracy theories. There was no one on the grassy knoll, no world government black helicopters, no alien lizard overlords. All very entertaining theories, but I think life shows us there are few conspiracies and a lot of cock-ups. On this issue, though, I really do wonder.

I suppose if any government came out and said, 'Hang on lads, we've screwed up, stop eating grains, stop eating low-fat spreads and skimmed milk and start eating more butter, lard, eggs and meat,' the consequences for all the industries that are behind those products would be potentially catastrophic. It would change farming and therefore the land and the environment.

The food processing industry is one of the biggest on earth. Naturally, it doesn't want us to stop eating processed food and start cooking for ourselves from separate ingredients now, does it? Of course not. Nor does it want us to eat less food. Less food means less profit. A fat dude is a profitable dude. Imagine if word got around that eating more fat stopped you getting as hungry and stopped you eating as much. It'd totally, well, knacker I think would be the technically correct economic term, all those industries that produce tasty little snacks to tide you over until your next big meal. Lots of money and lots of jobs rely on such industries.

Imagine what havoc would be wreaked on the grain industries if we all stopped, or even substantially reduced, eating bread and other grains. These industries are way too big and way too powerful to let this happen. That's what I'd think if I was a paranoid man. I'd think that they'd spend as much money as it took to persuade a lot of politicians, doctors and scientists to push the idea that whatever you made money from was essential for life itself and that not eating them will make the sky fall in. And I'd keep spending that money until the job was done.

If you're a government do you really want to push a message that might keep the population healthier but would also undoubtedly mean the collapse or decline of a lot of the food processing and agrarian industries which employ a lot of people and give up a lot of tax dollars? Probably not. There'd be all manner of wailing and gnashing of teeth from the rich and powerful grain lobby for a start – some of the most profitable land in the UK is dedicated to growing wheat – and those dudes ain't going down without a fight. A mass change in diet would put them out of business and create unemployment, at least in the short term.

But then again, if you've got land you can just grow something else, can't you? Perhaps not as profitably but all the same, a change in diet is an opportunity to do something different. But change is scary and the status quo guarantees big money. So no change is the preferred option.

The trouble is, we've got an economy that has become geared up to sell us utter shite. Take a look around your supermarket. Almost everything they sell is some sort of indulgence and far from being an essential foodstuff.

There's thirty foot of shelving dedicated to the all fat-inducing, no-nutrition, waste of money that is potato crisps. Another thirty foot dedicated to bloat-me-up-baby sugar and carb-packed biscuits and confectionery. Hey and how about another thirty foot full of bread products – how's your gluten intolerance doing? There's about double that dedicated to bloody breakfast cereals, all of which purport to be a healthy way to start the day but are little different to pouring milk onto chocolate biscuits or hob nobs. Just because it's got oats, dried fruit or 100 per cent of your daily fibre in it doesn't make it healthy.

Imagine all of those gone overnight, boom! Sorry, we don't need any of that crapola dude. 'Erk alors!' as the Lone Groover would have once said – one for the old *NME* readers there – because the fact is, this is all comedy comestibles; it's not freakin' food, man. It's in a supermarket but that doesn't make it food any more than the metal shelves it's sitting on. It's indulgence eating that has become so familiar, so everyday, that it's become an unthinking, massive part of most people's ordinary lives, and it's held in place by sheer volume of product and by constant advertising propaganda. Its constant presence invests these hugely contrived goods with an unremarkable ordinariness.

The one thing that all producers worry about is we the

customers. They worry we might stop being affected by their marketing and the prominent supermarket positioning of their stuff and start making up our own minds and walking away from their product. It scares them like daylight scares Dracula.

They can advertise it as much as they want and commission surveys or research to come up with the results they want to prove how great their products are but if the public are having none of it, if the public have chosen to walk a different path, there's sod all they can do. They're history. It might seem like they're almost above and beyond us, as though we're nothing to do with their continuation – especially when they've been around forever like Heinz Baked Beans or Kellogg's Cornflakes. But they all need our belief in them to keep going and they have to be in our face all the time for that to happen. They can't allow anything to be left unchallenged that suggests there's a good reason not to eat them.

When you or I talk about 'diet' we don't really connect what goes into our face with the global industry that came together to put it on the end of our fork or spoon. We have a vague idea, we get bits and pieces of info, but to piece it together into a complete planet-sized view of exactly how and why each thing has been grown, assembled, packaged, transported and sold is just too mind-blowing to get our head around. After all, it feels like we didn't really ask for all this to happen. It's just ... well ... there. And we buy it, thus justifying its existence, year after year. We went fairly blindly into this expansion of the processed food industry, being led by our appetite and our innate craving for a good time today, to eat and drink now for tomorrow we may die.

And that's how we went from a few hundred items being sold in a supermarket forty years ago to tens of thousands today. It's how we went from being a fairly lean country to being a nation of blubberhounds. We didn't mean to, honest. It just happened.

So no wonder that everyone who proposes a radically different way of eating, involving choices which totally by-pass much of the food industry, is often quickly painted as a quack, a nutter, a shyster. The way the food world is geared up to provide us with a starch-heavy, vegetable-oil-rich, intensively reared mass-produced meat diet has so become the norm that it's easy enough for the food industry to achieve this. The orthodoxy is so ingrained, the propaganda so deeply dug in. Any outsider looks wild and crazy. Look, all the doctors agree with us, they're educated and everything. Who are you to question them? You're a loony, a quack. There's the challenge.

At a time of unprecedented availability and diversity of food, so many of us, the majority of us, have lost the ability to think about food sensibly and rationally. We've become freaked out, perverted and paranoid about food.

Why don't we know what is best for us? Is it because at the core of our nature we are just self-destructive, live for now, monkey headbangers? Maybe this is just our destiny as a species. Maybe we'll never, en masse, break our short-termist, pleasure now, consequences later, mindset. And perhaps most radical of all, maybe it just doesn't really bloody matter. We live and we die. We leave little or no trace. Like my dad, just a small indentation on the sofa of existence. A cosmic blip of no consequence dedicated to killing ourselves to live.

Maybe. But as far as we know, we've only got one go at this existence game and it's so much more fun when you feel physically good and much less so when you don't. That's about as much as any of us can expect out of life and it's not such a big, ambitious dream. Some might say it should be the birthright for each and every one of us.

Fifty years ago my parents' generation were ambitious to change how and what they ate. They wanted to get away from their parents' old habits. They wanted to be more upmarket and more modern. They wanted to stop cooking so much and start heating up pre-made food. They wanted to buy their food in, not make it for themselves. The future was going to be clean and shiny. Take your protein pill and put your helmet on. What a beautiful world it will be, what a glorious time to be free.

Given where they had come from, it was understandable. It must have looked like progress but it is my view that it was an unmitigated disaster and set us on the road to our modern-day supermarket culture; a culture replete with processed and artificial food. It led to contrived foods seeming normal and natural food being too much trouble. It quite literally spoiled us.

Perhaps it was a journey that was inevitable. We had to see if the grass was greener on the other side of the food fence. It offered an easier life. It offered more pleasure and satisfaction for less money. It took the labour out of cooking. But we've seen what life is like when you give up eating simple, seasonal, natural ingredients. We've seen what happens when you surrender to processed, pre-made food; we've seen what all the new, modern foodstuffs have done to our physical and mental and even spiritual health.

So what the hell are we going to do? Massive global food empires have been created to thrust an almost infinite number of foods down our throats. We've lain back, opened up and swallowed. We've allowed them to make us compliant and allowed them to make us little more than gaping-mouthed saps, lapping up their advertising and marketing, unable to resist their honey trap of artificially sweetened, flavoured, value-added goodies. It's a way of life making so many of us fat and unhappy. We are eating ourselves into an early grave via a long and slowly debilitating decline. It's senseless.

It took fifty years to get here, but fifty years hence what will have become of us? Projections say that the vast majority of us will be obese and sick with Type 2 diabetes among many other lifestyle illnesses. We may have our lives extended by various pharmaceuticals and surgery, if we or the state can afford it, but the quality of our lives will have diminished even further. I'm not sure what more proof is needed that we have taken the wrong path. The evidence walks around us. Look what it did to me. If we keep on this track, blindly believing the one-size-fits-all healthy eating is always right and buying factory-made food and refusing to take responsibility for how we feed ourselves, it isn't going to end well.

It is as though we have become children and the food processing industry is our abusive parents. We just accept everything they push at us without question; we have surrendered our personal autonomy to this industry. We have whored ourselves to it and told them they can do what they want to us.

We have taken our hands off the wheel and are letting them crash the car. How many more metaphors do I have to write? We have to grow up, become adults and start looking after ourselves properly. There is nothing noble, clever or enjoyable about slowly becoming decrepit, about becoming fat, broke-down and unhappy.

We have to feed ourselves so that we don't fall ill but also so we can live life to the full and have a bloody good time. And the really stupid thing is, it is very, very easy to do – if we want to make the effort. And why wouldn't we want to make the effort?

But do we want to? Do we want to grow up and accept that discipline, personal responsibility and a basic understanding of food and cookery is something we owe to ourselves? If we don't, we won't deserve to live healthier, brighter, stronger and more content lives. I wanted to. I broke free from the hypnosis. It was one hell of a long fight and I damn near didn't make it. But it was one that I eventually won.

Things can be much, much better for us. A far better life was closer than I ever imagined it could be. When it comes to food, the choice is ours. It really is all up to us.

So what's it to be?

FURTHER READING

Allan, Christian B. and Lutz, Wolfgang, *Life Without Bread: How a Low-Carbohydrate Diet Can Save Your Life,* (McGraw-Hill Contemporary, 2000)

Blaylock, Russell L., *Excitotoxins: The Taste That Kills,* (Health Press, 1996)

Challem, Jack, *The Inflammation Syndrome: Your Nutrition Plan for Great Health, Weight Loss, and Pain-Free Living,* (John Wiley & Sons, 2010)

Daniel, Kaayla T., *The Whole Soy Story: The Dark Side of America's Favourite Health Food,* (New Trends Publishing Inc., 2009)

Enig, Mary and Falon, Sally, *Eat Fat, Lose Fat: The Healthy Alternative to Trans Fat,* (Plume, 2006)

Gittleman, Ann Louise, *Why Am I Always So Tired?,* (HarperOne, 2001)

Groves, Barry, *Trick and Treat: How Healthy Eating is Making Us Ill,* (Hammersmith Press Limited, 2008)

Ilardi, Dr Steve, *The Depression Cure: The Six-Step Programme to Beat Depression Without Drugs,* (Vermilion, 2010)

Schwarzbein, Diana, *The Schwarzbein Principle: The Truth About Losing Weight, Being Healthy and Feeling Younger,* (Health Communications, 1999)

Sears, Barry, *The Zone Diet,* (Thorsons, 2011)

Sisson, Mark, *The Primal Blueprint: Reprogram Your Genes for Effortless Weight Loss, Vibrant Health and Boundless Energy*, (Primal Nutrition Inc., 2009)

Sutter, Hannah, *Big Fat Lies: Is Your Government Making You Fat?*, (Infinite Ideas Limited, 2010)

Taubes, Gary, *Good Calories, Bad Calories: Fats, Carbs, and the Controversial Science of Diet and Health*, (Anchor Books, 2008)

Wilson, James L., *Adrenal Fatigue: The 21st Century Stress Syndrome*, (Smart Publications, 2002)

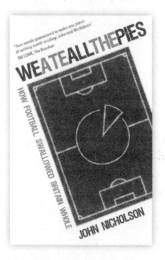